The Future of Biomedical Research

The Future of Biomedical Research

Claude E. Barfield and Bruce L. R. Smith, editors

AMERICAN ENTERPRISE INSTITUTE
and
THE BROOKINGS INSTITUTION
WASHINGTON, D.C.
1997

Available in the United States from the AEI Press, c/o Publisher Resources Inc., 1224 Heil Quaker Blvd., P.O. Box 7001, La Vergne, TN 37086-7001. Distributed outside the United States by arrangement with Eurospan, 3 Henrietta Street, London WC2E 8LU England.

AEI and Brookings wish to thank the Federation of American Societies for Experimental Biology for its support of this project. AEI also would like to thank the David and Lucile Packard Foundation and the Klingenstein Foundation for their support of the commissioned research papers.

Library of Congress Cataloging-in-Publication Data

The future of biomedical research / Claude E. Barfield and Bruce L. R. Smith, editors.
    p. cm.
    Includes bibliographical references and index.
    ISBN 0-8447-4036-5 (cloth).—ISBN 0-8447-4037-3 (paper)
    1. Medicine—Research—United States. 2. Medicine—Research—Government policy—United States. 3. Biology—Research—United States. 4. Biology—Research—Government policy—United States. I. Barfield, Claude E. II. Smith, Bruce L. R.
R854.U5F88   1997
610'.7'073—dc21   97-34604
                                              CIP

1 3 5 7 9 10 8 6 4 2

THE AEI PRESS
Publisher for the American Enterprise Institute
1150 17th Street, N.W., Washington, D.C. 20036

Printed in the United States of America

Contents

FIGURES

Contributors

CLAUDE E. BARFIELD has been a resident scholar and the director of science and technology policy studies at the American Enterprise Institute since 1983. Mr. Barfield was a consultant in the Office of the U.S. Trade Representative from 1982 to 1985. From 1979 to 1981, he was co-staff director and editor of the report of President Reagan's Commission for A National Agenda for the Eighties. Mr. Barfield has taught at Yale University, the University of Munich, and Wabash College. He has written and edited several books, including *Science for the Twenty-first Century: The Bush Report Revisited* (1997), *Technology R&D and the Economy* (1996, coedited with Bruce Smith of Brookings), and *Expanding U.S.-Asian Trade and Investment* (1997). He received his B.A. from Johns Hopkins University and his M.A. and Ph.D. from Northwestern University.

BRUCE L. R. SMITH retired from the Brookings Institution in 1996 after sixteen years as a member of its senior staff in the Center for Public Policy Education. Mr. Smith was a professor of public law and government at Columbia University from 1966 to 1979. While on leave from his university duties, and before joining Brookings, he was the director, Policy Assessment Staff, Bureau of Oceans, International Environmental and Scientific Affairs, in the U.S. Department of State. He lectures on recent trends in U.S. science policy, government-business relations, American politics, and other topics. Mr. Smith's scholarly publications include *Technology, R&D, and the Economy* (1996), with Claude E. Barfield, and *Sequencing? Financial Strategies for Developing Countries,* (1997). He received his B.A. *summa cum laude* and M.A. from the University of Minnesota. He was a Fulbright scholar in Germany, 1958–1959, and received a Ph.D. in government from Harvard University in 1964.

BRUCE ALBERTS is the president of the National Academy of Sciences. He was the chairman of the Commission of Life Sciences of the National Research Council and the president-elect of the American Society of Biochemistry and Molecular Biology. He is a principal author of *The Molecular Biology of the Cell*, a leading university textbook. Mr. Alberts has held positions at several colleges, including Princeton University and the University of California, San Francisco, where he was a professor and the vice-chairman of biochemistry and biophysics. He has been awarded an American Cancer Society Lifetime Research Professorship for work in biochemistry. Mr. Alberts's main focus has been the improvement of the teaching and learning process of the sciences at the elementary school level. He earned both his undergraduate and his doctorate degrees in biochemical sciences from Harvard University.

ALBERT A. BARBER is professor emeritus and past vice-chancellor of the University of California, Los Angeles. Mr. Barber was the chairman of the Zoology Department, vice-chancellor of research programs, and special assistant to the chancellor. He is a member of the American Association for the Advancement of Science, the American Physiological Society, and the American Society of Biochemistry and Molecular Biology. Mr. Barber lectures on university-industry relations, biomedical funding, and research animal use, as well as current and emerging issues in scientific research. He has served on numerous professional advisory committees and was the chairman of the board of the National Association for Biomedical Research and chairman of the California Biomedical Research Association. Mr. Barber has a B.S. and an M.S. from the University of Rhode Island and a Ph.D. from Duke University.

RALPH A. BRADSHAW is professor of physiology and biophysics at the University of California, Irvine, and the associate editor of the *Journal of Biological Chemistry and Growth Factors*. He was on the faculty of Washington University School of Medicine for thirteen years. Mr. Bradshaw has written nearly 300 scientific articles, with a concentration in the structure and function of proteins and a focus on polypeptide growth factors. He was the chairman of the U.S. National Committee for the International Union of Biochemistry and Molecular Biology and is a member and past chairman of the Executive Committee of the Keystone Symposia in Molecular and Cellular Biology. Mr. Bradshaw received his bachelor degree from Colby College and his doctoral degree from Duke University.

PURNELL W. CHOPPIN is the president of the Howard Hughes Medical Institute. He joined the institute in 1985 as vice-president and chief scientific officer, responsible for the major scientific programs of the Institute. At Rockefeller University, Mr. Choppin served as a professor, vice-president for academic programs, and dean of graduate studies. He headed the Rockefeller laboratory of virology, which concentrated on viral structure, replication, interaction with cell membranes, and the mechanisms by which influenza, parainfluenza, and measles viruses produce cell injury and disease. Mr. Choppin is a member of the National Academy of Sciences, American Academy of Arts and Sciences, and the Association of American Physicians. He has served on advisory groups for the American Cancer Society, the National Multiple Sclerosis Society, the Armed Forces Epidemiological Board, and the Scripps Clinic and Research Foundation. He was the chairman of the Memorial Sloan-Kettering Cancer Center from 1983 to 1984. Mr. Choppin received his medical degree from the Louisiana State University School of Medicine.

MICHAEL R. DARBY is the Warren C. Cordner Professor of Money and Financial Markets in the Anderson Graduate School of Management and the director of the John M. Olin Center for Policy in the Anderson School at the University of California, Los Angeles. He is the chairman of the Dumbarton Group, a research associate with the National Bureau of Economic Research, and an adjunct scholar with the American Enterprise Institute. Mr. Darby was the assistant secretary of the Treasury for economic policy, under secretary of commerce for economic affairs, and administrator of the Economics and Statistics Administration. He has written eight books and monographs and was the editor of the *Journal of International Finance*. Mr. Darby has served on the editorial boards of *American Economic Review, International Reports,* and *Contemporary Policy Issues.*

REBECCA S. EISENBERG is a professor at the University of Michigan Law School, where she teaches courses in patent and trademark law. She has written numerous articles on intellectual property issues in biomedical research, with particular attention to issues arising in the Human Genome Project. Ms. Eisenberg is studying how patents on DNA sequences affect technology transfer between the public and private sectors, under a grant from the U.S. Department of Energy.

MARK O. HATFIELD is a guest lecturer at George Fox University and Willamette University. He was the U.S. senator from Oregon, first elected in 1966. Mr. Hatfield was the chairman of the Senate Appropriations Committee and a member of the Energy and Natural Resources Committees, the Rules Committee, the Joint Committee on the Library, and the Joint Committee on Printing. He served two terms as governor of Oregon, from 1958 to 1966. Mr. Hatfield is the author of three books: *Not Quite So Simple* (1967), *Conflict and Conscience* (1971), and *Between a Rock and a Hard Place* (1976) and the coauthor of several others. Mr. Hatfield earned a B.A. from Willamette University and an M.A. from Stanford University.

ROBERT B. HELMS is a resident scholar and director of health policy studies at the American Enterprise Institute. He has written and lectured extensively on health policy, health economics, and pharmaceutical economic issues. Mr. Helms participates in the Consensus Group, an informal task force developing market-oriented health reform concepts. He is the editor of four recent AEI publications on health policy: *American Health Policy: Critical Issues for Reform; Health Policy Reform: Competition and Controls; Health Care Policy and Politics: Lessons from Four Countries;* and *Competitive Strategies in the Pharmaceutical Industry.* From 1981 to 1989, Mr. Helms was the assistant secretary for planning and evaluation and deputy assistant secretary for health policy in the Department of Health and Human Services. He holds a Ph.D. in economics from the University of California, Los Angeles.

R. GLENN HUBBARD is the Russell L. Carson Professor in Economics and Finance as well as the senior vice-dean of the Graduate School of Business at Columbia University. He is a research associate at the National Bureau of Economic Research, in programs on corporate finance, public economics, industrial organization, monetary economics, and economic fluctuations. He is also a visiting scholar at and adviser to the president of the Federal Reserve Bank of New York. Mr. Hubbard has taught at Northwestern University, the University of Chicago, and the John F. Kennedy School of Government. He has written more than seventy journal articles, edited several books, and written a leading textbook on money and banking. Mr. Hubbard has been an adviser or consultant to the Board of Governors of the Federal Reserve System, Congressional Budget Office, Internal Revenue Service, International Trade Commission, and the U.S. Departments of Energy and of Treasury. Mr. Hubbard's M.A. and Ph.D. in economics are from Harvard University and his B.A. and B.S. are from the University of Central Florida.

RICHARD A. JOHNSON is a senior partner in the Washington, D.C., law firm of Arnold & Porter. His practice specializes in international trade and technology matters. He was the general counsel for international trade at the U.S. Commerce Department. He also has served on numerous U.S. and international advisory groups concerned with trade, technology, and intellectual property issues and has testified before Congress about these matters. Mr. Johnson received a B.A. with highest honors from Brown University, an M.S. from the Massachusetts Institute of Technology, and a J.D. from Yale Law School.

ARTHUR KORNBERG is professor emeritus (active) of biochemistry at the Stanford University School of Medicine. He joined Stanford as the chairman of the biochemistry department in 1959. Mr. Kornberg had been a professor and the head of the microbiology department at Washington University School of Medicine. He was a researcher at the National Institutes of Health and a commissioned officer for the U.S. Department of Public Health. Mr. Kornberg is the author of several books, including *DNA Replication* (1980, 1992), *For the Love of Enzymes* (1989), and *The Golden Helix: Inside Biotech Ventures* (1995). He is a member of the National Academy of Sciences and the American Philosophical Society, a founder of the Policy Board, and a member of the Executive Committee and the Scientific Advisory Board of DNAX, a division of Schering-Plough Corporation. Mr. Kornberg has received several honors including the Gardner Foundation Award, the National Medal of Sciences, and the Nobel Prize in Medicine (with Dr. S. Ochoa) in 1959. He received his B.S. from City College of New York and his M.D. from the University of Rochester.

FRANK R. LICHTENBERG is Courtney C. Brown Professor of Business at the Columbia University Graduate School of Business and a research associate of the National Bureau of Economic Research. He has taught at Harvard University and the University of Pennsylvania. Mr. Lichtenberg worked at the Brookings Institution and was a visiting scholar at the Wissenschaftszentrum Berlin and the University of Munich. His research focuses on the introduction of new technology and its effects on the productivity of companies, industries, and nations and includes recent studies on the impact of new drugs on hospitalization rates and the effect of computers on productivity in business and government organizations. He has been awarded research fellowships by the National Science Foundation, the Fulbright Commission, and the Alfred P. Sloan Foundation and has been a consultant to private organizations and government agencies. Mr. Lichtenberg received a B.A. with honors in history from the University of Chicago and an M.A. and Ph.D. in economics from the University of Chicago.

CLARISA LONG is the Abramson Fellow at the American Enterprise Institute for Public Policy Research. Her research concerns the legal, economic, and policy issues surrounding intellectual property rights, genetic research, and the biotechnology industry. She was a molecular biologist at the Centre for Gene Technology in New Zealand and at the National Cancer Institute of the National Institutes of Health. The results of her scientific research have been published in the *American Journal of Kidney Disease, Cytokine,* and other publications. As an attorney in private practice, Ms. Long has prosecuted patents and worked on intellectual property, takings, and federal procurement cases. She served as a law clerk to Judge Alvin A. Schall of the U.S. Court of Appeals for the Federal Circuit. She has published in the *Stanford Law Review* and other scholarly journals and is a regular contributor to *Intellectual Property News.*

JUNE E. O'NEILL is the director of the Congressional Budget Office. She has been an economics instructor at Temple University (1965–1968), a research associate at the Brookings Institution (1968–1971), and a senior economist on the Council of Economic Advisers (1971–1976). She was the chief of the Human Resources Cost Estimates Unit at the Congressional Budget Office (1976–1979), senior research associate at the Urban Institute (1979–1986), and director of the Office of Policy and Research at the U.S. Commission on Civil Rights (1986–1987). In 1987, Ms. O'Neill became the director of the Center for the Study of Business and Government and professor of economics and finance at Baruch College and the Graduate Center at the City University of New York. She is also an adjunct scholar at the American Enterprise Institute. The author of many publications, Ms. O'Neill addresses the issues of income distribution, health insurance, labor supply and earnings, social security, welfare, and tax issues. She received her B.A. from Sarah Lawrence College and her Ph.D. from Columbia University.

HAROLD E. VARMUS is the director of the National Institutes of Health. He had been a professor of microbiology, biochemistry, and biophysics and the American Cancer Society Professor of Molecular Virology at the University of California, San Francisco. He and his UCSF colleague, J. Michael Bishop, shared a Nobel Prize in Physiology or Medicine in 1989 for demonstrating that cancer genes can arise from normal cellular genes, called proto-oncogenes. His research activities have assumed a special relevance to AIDS through a focus on biochemical properties of HIV and to breast cancer through the investigation of mammary tumors in mice. Mr. Varmus was the chairman of the Board of Biology for the National Research Council, an adviser to the Congressional Caucus for Biomedical Research, and cochairman of the New Delegation for Biomedical Research. He is the author or editor of four books and numerous scientific papers. Mr. Varmus received a B.A. from Amherst College, an M.A. from Harvard, and an M.D. from Columbia University.

PHILIP WEBRE is a senior analyst for the Natural Resources and Commerce Division of the Congressional Budget Office. He has written on science and technology issues for the CBO for over a decade and, together with others at CBO, has written several analyses of science budgeting. His most recent major publication, written with Judy Ruud of CBO, is *Emerging Electronic Methods for Making Retail Payments;* it analyzes proposed payment mechanisms for the Internet and stored-value cards. Mr. Webre's current research deals with other aspects of federal policy toward the Internet.

LYNNE G. ZUCKER is a professor of sociology, a professor of policy studies, and the director of the Organizational Research Program, Institute for Social Science Research, at the University of California, Los Angeles. She has worked as an economist with the Statistics, Income Division of the U.S. Internal Revenue Service. She also taught at the Department of Sociology at the University of Chicago and at the Ph.D. Program in Organizational Behavior at the Harvard Business School. Ms. Zucker has written four books and articles for journals on organizational theory, among them the *American Journal of Sociology* and *American Sociological Review.* She served on the NSF Young Presidential Scholar Award Panel and was the acting director of the UCLA Institute for Social Science Research.

1

Introduction

Claude E. Barfield and
Bruce L. R. Smith

The papers and commentary in this volume are the result of a productive collaboration of the American Enterprise Institute and the Brookings Institution with the Federation of American Societies for Experimental Biology. Aware of the growing list of complex issues that will challenge U.S. policymakers in the biomedical research and development area, FASEB asked AEI and Brookings to commission papers from leading academic researchers and top-level practitioners and to arrange a conference to analyze the findings before a broad audience from the science policy community, including members of Congress and their staff, administration officials, academics, and corporate executives from the biomedical sector. The papers were commissioned in the summer of 1996, and the conference took place in March 1997.

In remarks setting out the long-term issues facing the biomedical research enterprise in the United States, Harold Varmus, director of the National Institutes of Health, declared that the current period is "probably the most exciting time ever in the history of biology," citing the exploration of the blueprints of life in the genome project, studies in the neurosciences linking behavior to genetics, and the ability now to construct three-dimensional pictures of proteins and nucleic acids. These breakthroughs have built on the large-scale investments in the life sciences for the past five decades. Indeed, public and private support for R&D in the life sciences makes the field far and away the largest U.S. investment in a civilian research area.

In 1997, the United States will spend over $36 billion for biomedi-

1

cal research. This represents almost 20 percent of total U.S. R&D expenditures and about 40 percent of civilian R&D funding. For many years, the federal government footed most of the bill for research in the life sciences. Significant changes are taking place, however, and government dominance is no longer the case. Today, industry picks up 52 percent of the total R&D costs of health and biomedical research. NIH and other federal research programs account for just over a third of the total, with state and local governments at 6–7 percent, and nonprofit institutions at 4–5 percent. In 1997, the NIH budget totaled $12.7 billion.

The volume is organized as follows. In the opening overview section, leaders of American science, representing the federal government, the nation's top scientists, and the important foundation and nonprofit sector, present their views on the major policy questions in the life sciences. Among other issues, NIH Director Varmus highlights these challenges: the necessity to create mechanisms for stabilizing biomedical R&D funding; the need to ensure that research infrastructure—equipment and buildings—is adequate to support academic research; a clear assessment of the impact of the growing managed-care sector on research; balanced support for politically popular biomedical R&D with support for ancillary research areas that contribute key breakthroughs in medicine; a more rigorous system of research priority setting; and, finally, education of the public to the large societal payoff from biomedical and other research investments.

Bruce Alberts, National Academy of Science president, echoes some of Varmus's priorities, but he focuses on what he considers the urgent need to adapt graduate education in the biomedical and other sciences to current realities. Noting that "human capital is the most important product of the universities," he argues that leaders in the science community must ensure that the nation make better use of its young scientific talent. To achieve this goal, given the changing nature of future job markets, Alberts asserts that graduate education must broaden its focus to prepare students for a variety of careers—not just the narrow path toward tenure at a research university. He also urges universities to expand and deepen their guidance programs, citing his own contacts with students who "are confused" and "do not know what they want to do with their scientific skills."

Purnell Choppin, of the Howard Hughes Medical Institute, adds the perspective of the small but vital nonprofit biomedical research sector. He points to the major shift in the sources of support for biomedical research that has occurred over the past several decades—with industry now providing over half of the total. He argues that, even as the proportions of public and private support change, there is still a key role for the independent foundation and nonprofit support institutions. "One of the great strengths" of the U.S. system has been its pluralism, he states. The advantages that the nonprofit institutions bring to the process are flexibility and the ability to move rapidly into new scientific areas as opportunities develop, from the role of the Rockefeller Foundation in the 1920s to the Howard Hughes Institute and others today. They can also provide long-term support for individual scientists—something no other institution in the U.S. system can undertake—freeing them to concentrate on research without the necessity of endless paperwork and grant seeking.

The final contribution in the opening section is by a working scientist, Ralph Bradshaw, of the Department of Physiology and Biophysics, College of Medicine, University of California, Irvine. While he touches on some common problems of university-based research (such as the perennially vexing issue of indirect cost accounting), Bradshaw's chief concern relates to the current state of the peer review system, the process by which scientists' work is evaluated and rewarded (or not rewarded) with government or foundation research grants. He suggests reforms in the present peer review system to redress what he regards as biases against both young, entering researchers and senior scientists near the end of their careers.

The second major section of the volume examines the case for government support of basic research, particularly for support of biomedical R&D. Two different views of the nature of the science—and innovation—process and the underlying rationale for a government support system are presented. Nobel Laureate Arthur Kornberg, of Stanford University, argues forcefully that government science resource decisions should be made almost exclusively on the basis of scientific curiosity, and he is quite critical of disease-oriented research prioritization. He states that "the pursuit of curiosity about the basic facts of nature has proven throughout the history of medical science to be the most practical, the most cost-effective route to successful drugs and devices," and he points to a number of examples that support his assertion that "investigations that seemed totally irrelevant to any practical objective have yielded most of the discoveries of medicine." Moreover, Kornberg is fearful that the intermixing of research and commercial goals will have harmful effects, particularly for young scientists who may be seduced into pursuing "safe and practical projects over the untried and adventurous."

In direct contrast to Kornberg's arguments, Lynne Zucker and Michael Darby, of the University of California, Los Angeles, in their detailed analysis of the biomedical research field and of biotechnology commercialization, find a strong, positive synergy between scientific

3

achievement and financial and commercial goals. They argue that top-producing "star scientists" are the key to determining where and when private firms commercialize biomedical breakthroughs: the star scientists embody within themselves a "tacit knowledge" that even other scientists cannot fully comprehend; and, thus, they play a crucial role in technology transfer. Zucker and Darby also find that scientific productivity is enhanced by commercial collaboration; specifically, they demonstrate a direct correlation between patenting and commercial activity and increased publication and citation.

In his commentary on the two papers, Frank Lichtenberg, of Columbia University, finds himself not entirely comfortable with either view. He believes that Kornberg's arguments are politically naive and that public authorities will require some accountability from biomedical scientists for the use of public funds. Thus, he posits a middle way in which curiosity-based research can be augmented by disease-based allocation of R&D support, related to the relevant burden of the disease on society and to broader scientific opportunity. Conversely, Lichtenberg labels as "extreme" the Darby-Zucker view concerning the "natural excludability" of biomedical research discoveries.

Part three of the volume deals with long-term funding issues and the future support system for biomedical research. In the opening essay, Congressional Budget Office Director June E. O'Neill analyzes the implications for federal R&D spending of the commitment by the president and Congress to balance the budget by the year 2002. According to her calculations, discretionary spending—of which R&D is an important part—will decline 11 percent in real terms by 2002. While the fate of individual R&D programs cannot be predicted, O'Neill thinks that defense R&D is not likely to bear the brunt of funding cuts as it has in the recent past; thus, there will be greater pressure on civilian R&D programs, including biomedical R&D. Echoing Harold Varmus's warning, she cautions that, in deciding on cuts in spending, the nation should take care to maintain a "balance(d) . . . intellectual portfolio." Popular medical R&D programs should not be allowed to crowd out less politically powerful but still vital research in such areas as astronomy, chemistry, and physics.

In his commentary, Robert Helms, American Enterprise Institute, reinforces O'Neill's warning with a discussion of the growing demands on the federal budget from major entitlement programs, particularly Medicare and Medicaid. Drawing on his experience as a research administrator in the University of California system, Albert Barber describes the disparate impact that funding cuts by federal R&D agencies are likely to have on scientific disciplines and admonishes federal officials to avoid deep cuts in less well-known or politically appealing scientific disciplines. Again in contrast to Kornberg, Barber argues that the science policy community must tie its defense of public support for science more closely to societal goals and broad agency missions, such as the conquest of diseases, environmental cleanup, and weather prediction. "My thesis is simple," he states. "Basic research is strategic research."

The potentially negative consequences for biomedical R&D of a decline of federal discretionary funds have produced a search for more guaranteed funding stability. Among the ideas put forward has been the establishment of a dedicated trust fund for biomedical research, possibly financed from a tax on health maintenance organizations. In this section of the volume, the case for and the case against a biomedical trust fund are explored. Former senator Mark Hatfield (R.-Ore.) presents the arguments in favor of the proposal, and economist Glenn Hubbard from Columbia University, the arguments against the proposal. Hubbard contends that while there may well be a good case for maintaining or even increasing the level of support for biomedical research, a trust fund is not the best means to achieve this end.

In the final major section of the volume, Clarisa Long, from AEI, and Richard Johnson, from the law firm of Arnold & Porter, exhaustively analyze the complex emerging issues relating to intellectual property rights in biomedical research. They point out that the growing interface of the new genomics research field with intellectual property rights is already "profoundly reshaping the balance struck among the interests of biomedical research, private sector market participants and the public good." They discuss the controversy that has erupted in the wake of NIH's filing of applications for partial gene sequences, or expressed sequence tags (ESTs, in the biomedical lexicon). ESTs are short DNA sequences consisting of 150–400 base pairs. At the end of their essay, they conclude: "To date, the debate over the patentability of ESTs has centered on whether ESTs are patentable per se. The question that the intellectual property community and scientific community should focus on, however, is a different one: what scope of protection would be commensurate with the disclosed information?"

In her comments on that chapter, Rebecca Eisenberg, of the University of Michigan Law School, points out that what the Long/Johnson chapter describes is the growing privatization of biomedical research. By this she means that research that earlier would have been performed in the public sector and widely disseminated is increasingly likely to be performed in the private sector or privately appropriated as intellectual property by universities. Eisenberg expresses concern about important consequences of the privatization trend, particularly the potential for a creep of intellectual property protection into the upstream stages of biomedical research. Such a trend could hamper research and present major obstacles downstream by imposing burdensome licensing demands and expensive royalties on firms trying to bring pharmaceutical products to market. Given the diverse interests that must be accommodated—universities, NIH, small genomic firms, large pharmaceutical companies—together with the unstable legal framework, she concludes that the "task of putting together the bundle of intellectual property rights that are necessary to put new products on pharmacy shelves is costly and fraught with uncertainty."

These papers separately and collectively seek to define the major issues confronting the nation in ensuring continued U.S. leadership in biomedical research and in achieving the full social benefits of scientific advance. Biomedical research is both in a golden age of spectacular accomplishment and in a time of rapid change and instability. We hope that these essays will enrich the public debate on the critical issues and will contribute to a secure future for the biomedical research enterprise.

The editors would like to thank the staff of the Brookings Institution for the efficient handling of the administrative details of the March conference and the staff of the American Enterprise Institute for expediting the publication of this volume. In addition, Michael Jackson and Howard Garrison of the FASEB staff—as well as Ralph Bradshaw and John Suttie, who served as FASEB presidents during the project's inception and completion—provided invaluable advice and support.

PART ONE

Major Challenges for the Future

2

The View from the National Institutes of Health

Harold E. Varmus

This is a wonderful time for the National Institutes of Health, probably the most exciting time ever in the history of biology, with the exploration of the blueprints of life, the genomes of many organisms, including man; studies of neuroscience that are linking behavior to genetics; and the appreciation of life's images—from the three-dimensional structures of proteins and nucleic acids to pictures of organs that can be taken from outside the body.

I want first to comment on NIH funding, in view of the fact that NIH is the major supporter of biomedical research in the country. Then I will move beyond the obvious and necessary concern with annual appropriations to concentrate on nine long-term issues that have bedeviled me as NIH director and no doubt will bedevil those who think about the difficulties of supporting biomedical research and sustaining its integrity.

The NIH is a big player in the research game. We spent about 30 percent of the $36 billion the nation provided for health research and development in 1995. Industry, in the aggregate, picks up about 52 percent of the total R&D costs in the health arena. This is a change over the past ten years. In 1986, NIH supported 42 percent of health R&D, whereas industry provided less, 38 percent. There are other significant players but on a much smaller scale—federal sources other than the NIH account for about 10 percent; state and local sources, around 6–7 percent; and nonprofit organizations, around 4–5 percent. The current

9

NIH budget is $12.7 billion. We have had modest but significant and encouraging increases over the past several years, particularly for the last two years, in which budgets have been cut for many federal agencies. Strong support in Congress accounts for healthy increases of 6 percent and almost 7 percent for NIH in difficult budgetary times. Of that $12.7 billion, roughly 85 percent is spent to provide extramural support to investigators all over the country in over 2,000 different institutions. About 10 percent goes to support of the NIH intramural research program. The money is appropriated directly to more than 20 institutes and centers, which have budgets that range from roughly $20 million to over $2 billion. About 57 percent of NIH's money is spent on research project grants. Other expenses include contract programs, administrative costs, and the intramural program. Our prospects for the coming year look quite good; we are encouraged by statements from a number of our supporters in Congress. The president has requested a 2.6 percent increase for NIH, and we will likely end up doing somewhat better than that.

But moving beyond these annualized funding figures, I will discuss nine other issues to set the stage for a broad consideration of what is needed over the long haul to sustain the vitality of what we do. The first four of these nine admittedly require money in some form but in a somewhat different guise than the traditional annualized appropriations.

The first of these issues is the need to find some means to stabilize the funding situation. One of the problems we have as administrators of federal funds for research is that the NIH as an institution gives out multiyear awards for many long-term activities and yet is supported by annual appropriations. This means that the NIH has a large commitment base; probably close to 85 percent of our money is in the commitment base. This has a major effect when we are threatened with short-term budget cuts.

The threat to NIH support for fiscal year 1996, for example, is well known; it was argued that all federal agencies should take cuts as part of the national resolve to balance the budget. But a 5 percent or 10 percent cut in NIH funding would have meant few or no new grants unless we lowered the amount we provided for those to whom we had already made long-term commitments.

What are the options for sustaining a more stabilized funding pattern? There have been many suggestions, none of them totally satisfactory for political or operational reasons. One possibility is an appropriations process that allows us to use the money given to us in any single year over the several years of a grant. I am worried about this approach. What we have works fairly well, and I am not sure I want to make such a radical change. There is also much talk about trust funds. While I applaud that idea, many people resist it as just another tax. And if one institution has a trust fund, everyone else will clamor for a trust fund—where will it stop? There is also the possibility of stabilizing the situation by tapping other sources of funding: donations, partnerships with voluntary organizations—we have some, but they do not provide a large amount of money in relation to our total funding pool; and royalties for inventions—a nice idea, but we recoup only about $20 million a year through royalties, and that will not have a major effect. So these are unresolved problems.

The second issue is our need to adapt to changes in health care reimbursement. Although I am tired of this topic, it is impossible to ignore its effects. A large fraction of biomedical research is done at academic health centers, and there is a large effect on academic health centers brought about by the enlargement of the managed-care industry. We have had a hard time determining exactly what the fiscal effect is, but it is probably a loss of revenue in the range of $1 billion a year. How do we deal with this problem? I have been speaking with managed-care organizations about common research interests in the hopes of achieving opportunities for cofunding of the research that we are mutually interested in. These activities may happen. Speaking with the more enlightened members of what is definitely a heterogeneous group of corporations, we are finding some managed-care organizations that are quite sympathetic to working jointly with the academic health centers to do research. But any activities that ensue will likely be confined strictly to areas of mutual interests—activities that account for less than a third of our current expenditures. We have some models for how this might work, based on interactions among federal agencies. The National Cancer Institute and the Department of Defense, for example, have been working together to fund the clinical costs of military patients in NCI's sponsored trials through the Civilian Health and Medical Program for the Uniformed Services (CHAMPUS) Tricare program of the DOD. A large-scale clinical trial organized by the Heart, Lung, and Blood Institute is being supported by Medicare. These arrangements provide potential models for how interactions with the managed-care industry might work.

The third issue is how to ensure the vitality of the research infrastructure. Buildings, equipment, and support for training are vital to the long-term viability of the research establishment but are the part of the enterprise that is under the most stress in times of fiscal stringency. When growth is relatively slow, our tendency is to support grants rather than support buildings. That is the right decision year by year, but, at some point, it takes its toll. One of the major issues that

11

face us as administrators of federal funds for research is how to gauge when the infrastructure is, in fact, unduly frayed and when we should be stepping in. Who makes those decisions? Should we leave them up to the institutions in which erosions of infrastructure are occurring? Or should we have a national commission that says an institution now needs additional support to restore its facilities or to acquire additional equipment? And how much should we spend as a federal partner in this arrangement to repair things?

The fourth issue is how to promote a sometimes frayed set of intersections between the government and academia or between the government and industry. There is a long laundry list of things that we are trying to do to make sure that those important intersections are as smooth as possible. We have programs to encourage the sharing of resources between the industrial sector and the academic or government sectors through small business innovation grants and cooperative research and development agreements. We also have a continuing problem with indirect cost reimbursement and how we set rates. The Office of Management and Budget is working on a new set of rate determination guidelines, which we hope will improve the way in which we do business. We have a long-standing debate with the academic sector about the best way to reimburse tuition costs; we have made some improvements here, but they are not totally satisfactory. We are also concerned about what happens when established investigators lose their grants because competitive renewal applications do not score well. We have tried to institute awards to give investigators at least some support for another year while their renewal applications are being rewritten and rereviewed. That program has been somewhat successful, though it is not a complete cure for the problem. We have tried to develop better ways of communicating with our grantees, especially in academia. Electronic communication has successfully cut the cost of our interactions, but use is still quite limited in scope.

The other five issues I would like to discuss involve the conduct of science and modes of advocacy or of policy. These boil down to matters of conviction rather than matters of finance.

One thing that has concerned me over the past several years is determining the steps that we can take to guarantee that science, including medical science, is perceived by the public and Congress as a field that is equitable and has a high level of integrity. There is a range of issues here, and I cannot touch on them all. One issue is how we can be more effective in recruiting minorities into science. We have not been especially successful in this area. I am still concerned about the low level of representation of Hispanic and African-American scientists in our culture; we need to seek better ways to improve this. A perennial problem for us has been how we deal with allegations of misconduct and how we judge instances of fraud. We have made some progress in the past few years. The federal government as a whole, through the National Science and Technology Council and through the NIH and the Department of Health and Human Services, in particular, has worked hard in recent months on developing new definitions and guidelines regarding misconduct. Some of them will be announced soon.

The sixth issue concerns how we resolve disputes over technology transfer and patent rights. I see an increasing tendency to emphasize reach-through rights rather than one-time fees when negotiating licenses for items such as pieces of DNA, transgenic animals, or other items that are used in research. When such research tools are licensed with reach-through rights, there are consequent disincentives to develop products and possibly strong disincentives to do the research that is required to develop them. In a recent address, an official of the Patent and Trademark Office claimed that the PTO has made a decision to consider the patenting of expressed DNA sequences on the basis that there is utility in using these sequences as molecular probes. Exactly how that kind of patent would be issued—what rights would be given to the patent holder—is not yet known. This is a decision that we are likely to contest publicly.

The seventh issue is how we improve the dividends that we get from our research dollars. Everyone in this fiscal era is concerned about efficiency, and we are thinking about many different ways to approach the question of how we get more return on dollars invested. One thing we have always prided ourselves on at NIH is peer review, but we also recognize that peer review is an imperfect process. We have a new director of our Division of Research Grants, Elvira Ehrenfeld, who is mounting an effort to align our study sections properly with current areas of biomedical research and to improve the peer review process. We also need to be more rigorous about priority setting. We need to explain to the public and Congress how we make our judgments and also face the fact that this is a process with subjective components. Another need is to diversify the areas of research that are currently pursued, particularly by our new grantees, who often have just emerged from the most active areas of science and are most likely to continue with them. How long can we allow such fields to increase in size at the expense of other fields that might not attract as many new trainees?

In other efforts to promote efficiency, we need to hold down the costs of certain active research disciplines. This matter has come frequently to my attention in recent weeks because we at NIH are focusing on initiatives to maximize the outcome per dollar when developing animal models. We need better means to govern the costs of animal experiments, whether this involves cost sharing with universities, rate setting for facilities costs, or other ways to support jointly the cost of animal research. A better sharing of resources, databases, and informatics and a streamlining of the regulatory apparatus may all be important.

The eighth issue is particularly important for a group focusing on biomedical research. Those of us who support biomedical research—an intrinsically popular field of research because of its health benefits—need to be reminded that our research is dependent on many other allied disciplines. Those disciplines include chemistry, math, physics, computer science, and social science. All these other sciences are much more vulnerable to the severe consequences of eroding support in a fiscally limited world. In our work at the NIH, we have seen the tremendous impact of chip-based informatics that are used in nucleotide sequencing; of laser technology in strategies that range from clinical treatments to karyotyping; of the use of structure-based drug design. These methods all depend heavily on principles of physics, math, and computer science—disciplines that are jeopardized because we are training too few people in those fields and offering too few opportunities, because we are focusing too narrowly on the biological aspect of medical science and not recognizing the importance of other disciplines in building the infrastructure.

The last item is the need to convince the public, Congress, and the administration that medical research has many benefits, not simply the ever-popular prospect of living longer and living healthier. These are important goals, but there are many others. The traditional alternative goals involve the prospects of saving costs through the prevention of illness or its complications or through cheaper treatment. Our research does increase expenses in certain cases, but we effect cost-savings in others. Another traditional means of convincing people of the benefits of medical research is to point out the effect of that research on science education. Some of the discoveries and developments in medical research are exciting to teach to students and can encourage them to enter scientific careers. We scientists take pride in the national esteem that comes from our discoveries and from our world leadership in the area of biomedical research. We are also proud that we stimulate many industries, most obviously the biotechnology and pharmaceutical industries. These are among the traditional benefits that we can point to.

Two other possibilities could have a major effect on the way in which the nation thinks about medical research. The first is the possibility of improving international relations through the use of science, in particular biomedical science, as a means to recognize global closeness and the necessity of nations to work together. I offer as one example the effort that the NIH has made through the National Cancer Institute to promote a Middle East Cancer Consortium. This effort provides one of the few vehicles that allow representatives of the states of the Middle East to sit down at a common table and talk about common interests. There are other ways in which we might promote better international relations using our concern for scientific questions that can be addressed in a multilateral fashion, and medical research again offers particularly useful examples.

The second point is the potential for using medical research as a means to achieve political stability in many parts of the world. Some may have read a recent story by Jeffry Goldberg in the *New York Times Sunday Magazine* about the destabilizing effects of AIDS, malaria, and tuberculosis on African politics. I recently spent a couple of weeks in West Africa looking at the impact of malaria on the economies and politics of two countries. All of us who have seen what AIDS is now doing to Asia have recognized the importance of achieving better prospects for health to avoid the chaos that has occurred in many parts of Africa. Emphasizing international issues can also help diversify our science by drawing students to problems that are slighted in current biomedical research in this country. And it can help to recruit additional funds—for example, by encouraging all governments, not just ours, to recognize that medical research is a potentially stabilizing influence.

3

The View from the National Academy of Sciences

Bruce Alberts

I will focus on only one part of a complex system, but it is the part most essential when focusing on the health of the enterprise and its future: the young people who are now graduate students and postdoctoral fellows coming up through the system who will be the next generation of biomedical researchers, scientists in various policy positions, and leaders in many other places in society. I have been asked to review many different institutions; I have done more such reviews than I would like to admit. But I always try to concentrate on this simple issue. Is the institution that I am reviewing—whether it is intramural NIH, a university department, or a private research institute—taking in as their new researchers, some of the best young people in the world? And is the institution supporting them in ways that will allow them to be successful and productive?

One could look at many other things. One could look at citation indexes, publication lists, society memberships, and so on to evaluate a research organization. But the easiest thing to measure is what I measure, and it really is the right indicator for the future vitality of the institution.

Since I have been president of the National Academy of Sciences, I have been asked to speak to many different graduate student groups. It is important for people like me to get out of my office and beyond the beltway to meet with graduate students. Most recently, I spent a whole day, ending at midnight, with about four hundred graduate students in the biomedical sciences at Yale. These students had organized an all-day-Saturday affair, where they presented some of their best research and talked about some of their aspirations and goals. I have also met with many other graduate student groups in the past few years.

The good news is the tremendous amount of talent among the young people coming up through the system who want to be biomedical scientists. They are able, energetic, motivated. They are terrific people with high standards and good values. They are being well educated and well prepared. Certainly, they know much more at their age than I did. And the average quality of students at our leading institutions actually is higher than when I was a graduate student. They also, it seems, are quite willing to do almost anything for a career that makes use of their scientific talents in productive ways.

I attended the first graduate student fair that focused on careers for future graduate students—a famous one held about three years ago at Stanford University. Initially only a small number was expected, but this discussion of the future for students in the biomedical sciences was so popular that it filled one of the largest auditoriums at Stanford. In the end, young people were busing into Stanford from all over the Bay area for an all-day, standing-room-only session. That was the wake-up call for some of us older scientists that there was a real need for better communication with students. At that meeting, one could immediately sense a feeling of hostility in many of the young people. They felt that they had been misled because they had been told that there could be a shortage of scientists by the time they entered the job market. But now it was clear that there would not be nearly enough research jobs.

More recently, at similar meetings, I find that the attitude has completely changed. Young people are flexible. What I hear repeatedly is that they are not fixed on a research career anymore. They have adjusted quite rapidly to the idea that they may not be a professor, may not have an independent research group. But they want to find something useful to do with their scientific talents—a career in which they can be productive and contribute to the general scientific enterprise.

So all that is good news. The bad news is that we have not done a good job of making career options clear for them. Meanwhile, a National Research Council study showed, over a year ago, that the population of independent investigators in the biological sciences is aging considerably. The council has a follow-up study that will appear later this year. It traces where all the young biological scientists who are not becoming independent investigators at a young age are going.

I was an assistant professor at the age of twenty-eight, which was typical in 1966. Whereas I spent one-year as a postdoctoral fellow, now people hang around for five or even ten years in such postdoctoral positions. At least part of the reason for the aging of independent researchers is the much higher threshold: one needs to be almost internationally famous as a researcher with many publications to get a position as an assistant professor these days. I would never have been offered my position in 1966 with such a requirement. So the age at which scientists are becoming truly independent is going up, and that is unfortunate for many reasons. People are creative and energetic at young ages, and it is important for the success of this enterprise that we try to provide our best people with the independence that allows them to try out their own ideas as soon as possible.

The other part of the bad news is that there are many young people who do not know what they want to do with their scientific skills. These scientists are confused, and they need guidance. Unfortunately, most faculty members cannot provide this guidance for them. Most of my colleagues do not know anything about careers other than being a professor. Before I came to Washington, I was also handicapped in this way.

Thus, even though faculty want to help their students, they are not doing a good job of advising them. And we badly need to outgrow the traditional attitude that those students and postdoctoral fellows who are not going to become professors are failures. The old attitude in my field was that if a young scientist went to industry, that was a failure—if he or she did anything else, God forbid. Only those who became professors, and particularly professors at certain schools, were viewed as really successful. Today, such an attitude is totally destructive of the enterprise. If we do not change our narrow view of success and if we fail to convey our support for many other careers for our students, both science and the nation will suffer.

Even in biology, where the fraction of our doctorates going into academic careers has traditionally been highest, not much more than one-third of these people are today finding academic career pathways available to them.

The National Research Council and the academies have been trying to do our part to encourage our young people and provide them with better advice. We have, for example, prepared a special career guide for students, which is being widely used. This guide elaborates a range of career options, and it is freely available on the World Wide Web associated with an electronic site that aims to connect an inquiring student to an actual person who can give them advice on whatever career they are exploring (www.nap.edu/readingroom/books/careers). We hope that we can help our young people head toward the right places, both those who want to do research and those who do not want to do research. The next step in this effort, which is about to come out, is a mentoring guide designed to help faculty become better advisers for young scientists.

This brings us to the whole question of what type of graduate education is optimal. In April 1995, the academies released a major report entitled *Reshaping Graduate Education for Scientists and Engineers*, which emphasizes the need to prepare students for a wider variety of career options. Talking with people in industry makes clear that the most important product of research at universities is the human capital, the students whom we are educating. Our report includes a suggestion that graduate students, sometime during their Ph.D. study, spend several months somewhere else—in industry, in Washington working on science policy, in a local office of the Environmental Protection Agency, or a place that uses science in other ways—and then come back to complete their research.

Because anything that one graduate student knows all the graduate students know, the net result of all these outside experiences would be a much greater familiarity with a range of career options for all students. Students will finish a Ph.D. in five years more often if they actually know what they want to do next, rather than feeling that they need to hang around because they do not know any other option than trying for an academic position.

Finally, I want to discuss the intellectual problem, which I have been worried about for many years but is only getting worse. There are tremendous opportunities in biology today. I am a molecular and cell biologist, and my students know a lot of fundamental things about cells. They could work on any human biology problem or on plant biology. The tools that they have need to be applied very broadly. The trouble is that many of our most talented young people want to do something that is exciting and new in research for their career, but they do not have diverse enough models: they have only their professors. Too often they try to do exactly what we do. And, as a result, perhaps fifty people publish about the Ras protein every month, and almost nobody works on the crucial question of why bone tissue grows when it is subjected to pressure.

Many tremendously interesting and important problems are not being addressed by modern techniques. There is no real wake-up call to the young people that these problems exist and that they can be attacked only by the methods and the skills that they have. And here is a real obligation and an opportunity for us older scientists to try to help young people come to grips with the tremendous intellectual challenges in biology and in biomedical science, in particular. How can we do a much better job, for example, of connecting to clinical

19

departments, where there are so many wonderful biological problems of both theoretical and practical importance that clinicians do not have the tools to address?

Our culture needs to change in some way. I am interested in trying new kinds of experiments. Could we set up something that is more collaborative than the typical university research program? Could we develop a new role for small groups of senior faculty, in which they would facilitate the work of younger scientists, serving as mentors who encourage new creative kinds of biomedical science without putting their names on the resulting papers as authors? Since everyone wants to get credit for the things that they do, could there be a special kind of recognition for such service that distinguishes it from regular authorship?

I do not know the answer to these questions, but I believe that the community should try to establish new models to complement our traditional ways of doing research. This is an important challenge to all of us who occupy responsible leadership positions.

4

The View from the Howard Hughes Medical Institute

Purnell W. Choppin

As a representative of a large not-for-profit funder of biomedical research, my discussion reflects a point of view from the private not-for-profit sector. But I hasten to add that, for most of my professional career, I was a research scientist funded by generous grants from the NIH and also from the National Science Foundation and, occasionally, from private not-for-profit sources.

Like Dr. Varmus and Dr. Kornberg, I want to emphasize briefly the fact that we are in a revolutionary time in terms of the opportunities for biomedical research. Dr. Kornberg said that "the future is in the headhunting side of the game." Phil Sharp, one of our good friends, in looking at the future of research, has said, "We are now formulating the concepts of how we formulate concepts." This is an interesting way of looking at neuroscience research.

My point of view, as a not-for-profit funder, on some of the challenges that are facing long-term research is no different from the others. But I would like to start with a general challenge, an anonymous quotation that I read some years ago in a conservation magazine: "We don't inherit the land from our parents; we borrow it from our children." We can use a similar analogy in biomedical research: We in our generation cannot simply profit by the remarkable advances that have been made by our predecessors and by our contemporaries, but we must do everything we can to expand knowledge to the fullest extent possible and guarantee our children and their children the ability to reap the benefits of what we do today. I mean not only continuing research but also making sure that we have the next generation of scientists through training and education today to continue the revolution tomorrow.

Harold Varmus has addressed most of the issues that I would mention as challenges, but I will briefly continue the theme he began. That is, we have discussed mostly the continued challenge of investing in research, and I mean the word *investing* in every sense. We must sustain these wonderful advances, and that is a tall order when we hear about what is happening to discretionary funding. But, in some sense, that might be easier than some of the other challenges, so long as we have people such as Congressman Porter and Senators Specter and Harkin and former senator Hatfield, as champions.

But what we have to do also is to continue to produce the next generation of scientists. That not only means funding their training, but it means convincing the best and the brightest that there will be careers in the long-term future and careers in which they will be supported. That is an increasingly difficult task when they see their current mentors and mentors-to-be spending such a tremendous amount of time seeking support for doing research. That is a challenge that we have to face, one that is beyond the immediate funding problem.

Finally, we must do what we can to ensure that the institutions that are carrying out most of the biomedical research in this country—and, by that, I mean the academic medical centers and the great research universities—are still there, healthy and vigorous, to carry out that research. Much has been said about the impact of managed care on the academic health centers, and Harold Varmus discussed the large amount of the money from patient care revenues going into research that is being eroded. He used a term of *a billion*. Some estimates are even higher than that. But it is a large sum and it is being eroded. Even 6.5 percent increases in the NIH budget, let alone 2.6 percent increases, cannot make up the deficit that is being created in the revenues of these centers. We simply have to find some way to support them.

The final word on that point comes from Abraham Flexner, who wrote in 1910 the Flexner Report, which revolutionized medical education and ultimately medical research in this country. His main point in that report is that the medical schools at the time were overly commercial, and they were divorced from an academic and scientific background. If we do nothing to stop the trend that is being forced on the medical schools because of managed care, in 2010 we will need another Flexner Report that tries to salvage a system that is now the envy of the world but in grave danger.

In 1979, the federal government provided 69 percent of the biomedical research and development in this country, and industry provided 29 percent. By 1994, the federal government was providing 37 percent, and industry, 52 percent. Now industrial support for biomedical research is not bad—it is good. I wish there were more of it. But these are R&D numbers—and industry is much more likely to be D and the federal government is much more likely to be R. One cannot escape the conclusion that the proportion of basic research in this country has been going down over the past fifteen years.

Now what about the private, not-for-profit support? Interestingly enough, in 1930, private, not-for-profit support of medical research equaled federal support. By 1940, in just ten years, private, not-for-profit support was only 27 percent of the total, and, by 1980, it was less than 4 percent, and that is where it has remained. Today, 3.7 percent of the total biomedical R&D dollars is being provided by the private, not-for-profit sector.

I am both pleased and concerned to say that if it were not for the rapid increase in the spending of the Howard Hughes Medical Institute, the number would not be 3.7 percent; it would be 3 percent. One institution is now providing over 20 percent of the total private, not-for-profit support in medical research.

One of the strengths of this country has been not only what the federal government has provided and what industry has provided but the pluralism that has also been made possible by private, not-for-profit support.

I hope that will continue. Recently, some large foundations and wealthy individuals have begun to put more money into the biomedical research sphere. The health of the biomedical research enterprise, however, is inexplicably tied to that of the federal government now.

What are some advantages of private, not-for-profit support? Flexibility is probably the greatest advantage, the ability to move rapidly into a new area and, conversely, the ability to stay with a given area of research, even though results are not forthcoming rapidly.

One can take an individual approach to support the career of an individual or take an institutional approach, which is sometimes difficult for the federal government to do. One can support the careers of scientists rather than taking a project-based support, whereas government support understandably is predominantly project based because of the way the money is largely appropriated. Private support can take the other course, that is, supporting careers on a long-term basis.

And, finally, private sources can use their resources to complement government efforts. In my organization, we try to do that, to complement the NIH. We are not only located just down the road from the NIH in Chevy Chase, Maryland, but we cooperate directly in a num-

23

ber of efforts. The Howard Hughes Medical Institute, as the name implies, was founded by Howard Hughes in 1953.

Interestingly, he put the words *basic research* into the charter of the institute. He was concerned, in his own words, that the institute be involved in trying to understand the genesis of life processes. And so *basic research* has remained in our charter since the beginning.

In 1984, a new board of trustees was appointed and sold the only asset of the institute, the Hughes Aircraft Company, which Howard Hughes had given to the institute in 1953, when he founded it. We have been in the enviable position of having our budget increase ninefold since 1984. The sale of the aircraft company was at a remarkably good time, and the stock market has been good to the institute, so that its budget is now $455 million per year—and more than 80 percent of that supports medical research.

HHMI is not a foundation. It is something called a medical research organization, which means that we directly support research by investigators who become our employees, even though they are faculty members in medical schools and research universities around the country. We now have over 300 such laboratory heads in approximately 70 institutions around the country. We enter into close, collaborative arrangements with the institutions where our investigators are faculty members. We provide their full salaries as well as research support.

In 1987, as a result of an enlightened agreement with the Internal Revenue Service, we became able to spend money not just to support research of our investigator-scientists but to become involved in science education. We are doing that at the level of about $86 million a year. That is science education at every level, from elementary school through college undergraduate, predoctoral, and postdoctoral fellowship programs.

The institute is involved in education with two goals: to make sure that we have the next generation of well-trained scientists and to try to raise the level of scientific literacy in the general population. In a democracy, all the money ultimately comes from the people, and they need to be informed in order to make their own decisions about how the budget should be deployed.

My institution has been fortunate to be active at a time when the science advances are so rapidly forthcoming. HHMI has been able to identify some of the best and brightest scientists. We ask of them a minimum amount of paperwork. We support their careers over long terms and, periodically, we review them rigorously to confirm that they are still doing outstanding research, but in the interim they are free to schedule their own work. The results speak for themselves. Five of them are Nobel Prize winners and over sixty are members of the National Academy of Sciences. In 1994, the Institute for Scientific Information reported that 25 percent of all the so-called hot papers in biology in that year were authored by HHMI scientists. I am also happy to say that this year we intend to increase the number of scientists who we are supporting by about 25 percent, an action made possible by the increase in our endowment.

5

The View from a Working Scientist

Ralph A. Bradshaw

The challenge to generate the resources to support scientific research, and in particular biomedical research, at a level that will sustain the growing momentum since the end of the Second World War will be a major priority of government, business, and academia for the new millennium. There is an interdependent relationship between the three, with a role for each, and each must fulfill this role if the promises of better health and improved quality of life that have become increasingly expected by the public are to be realized. Thus, government must continue to provide the support for basic research, and companies must continue to invest funds through their extensive development programs to see that the new knowledge generated will eventually become new products, such as medicines and treatments. At the same time, academia must maintain its productivity through wise deployment of the available resources. It is not inappropriate to consider briefly what it can do to improve on its part in this three-way partnership, even as both government and industry are prodded to increase their commitments.

The university or research institute is an essential component in the biomedical research enterprise, providing the environment and infrastructure for scientists to carry out their basic work and, at the same time, providing for the training of the next generation of investigators. The well-being of our higher education system cannot be overstressed in any discussion of expanding support for research. Educational issues are sometimes seen as being at cross-purposes with research and often suffer (or receive less attention), particularly at larger, research-oriented campuses. These problems have to do with prestige and the emphasis that faculty and staff place on research when making decisions regarding advancement and are usually related to fiscal issues, that is, the internal distribution of funds. Since it is not always easy to separate the expenses of pedagogical and research activities, university faculty and administrators are faced with a financial balancing act on a regular basis. In public institutions, departmental budgets, invariably provided to support only teaching, can be totally inadequate to maintain even minimal services, and additional money must be generated to make up this difference. This often comes from research-related activities. This situation creates an interesting paradox: faculty are personally rewarded for their research accomplishments, while their departments receive no institutional fiscal recognition or return for these same endeavors.

Nowhere is this problem more acute than in the handling of indirect costs, those moneys paid to universities and institutes to provide infrastructure and support for research. The extent to which these are really used to support research as opposed to maintaining other academic functions (including a generally perceived ballooning bureaucracy) has been extensively discussed and debated and remains an important issue. On the one hand, savings in these costs should eventually mean increased dollars for direct costs; on the other, inappropriate changes could severely damage universities and institutes, with concomitant negative effects on the instructional functions that are essential to the educational structure of the country. Thus, solving problems, such as those created by excess regulation, is an immediate way to increase grant dollars without any increase in budget or any adverse impact on other parts of the academic enterprise, but indiscriminate cuts or caps could be devastatingly destructive.

At the same time, university administrators need to be mindful that simply passing on research costs to investigators that should properly be paid by institutions is equally damaging to investigative activities. The best indicator of research effectiveness is not total dollars or even the number of research grants—it is the number of people actually working at the bench. That is where the data are collected, and data are the heart of new information. This parameter reveals whether research is growing, shrinking, or staying the same. Although calculations based on buying power, inflation, or other financial indicators may be satisfying to economic analyzers of science, they are, at best, indirect measures of the research enterprise. Every time a stipend for a student or postdoctoral fellow or a salary for a technician is lost to pay for waste disposal or increased animal care, science contracts even though the dollar amounts stay the same.

Peer Review

While the foregoing remarks suggest that the funds already awarded for research might be better managed internally in institutions, the distribution of this same research moneys at the agency level—based on peer review evaluations—remains a matter of substantial concern. This is a scientist-based issue and is no less difficult to deal with than regulation or indirect costs and is no less destructive to the research community. The problem can, in fact, be couched in the same terms that have been effectively used to lobby Congress as to why it is so damaging to cut funds for biomedical research; that is, a research program builds momentum through creating a body of knowledge, along with a trained group of workers, and when grants are cut off, the program terminates, workers disperse, and the incomplete research efforts are largely, if not completely, lost. Only after others have repeated much of the same work can the thread usually be picked up again, with considerable time and money wasted on redundant efforts. Thus, when a senior investigator loses funding, there is not only a loss of knowledge but also the loss of experience and accumulated wisdom, which cannot be directly replaced. The situation is equally damaging when a beginning investigator is involved. Despite no loss of an existing program and amassed information, no hierarchical structure such as the academic research community can afford to deny entry to the young scientists who will become tomorrow's senior investigators. Hence, no process has a greater effect on research than the rating of grant proposals.

Although peer review takes many forms in science, it is always characterized by certain guiding principles. First and foremost, it assumes, as the name implies, that the judges are the equals, or peers, of those being judged. Second, this review assumes a code whereby those with a vested interest in the decision, for whatever reason, will excuse themselves from the deliberation and decision and that the material under consideration will not be used inappropriately or abused. Finally, it requires a spirit of collegiality, a commitment to the advancement of science, which manifests itself in decisions that are unbiased by real or perceived prejudices about individuals, institutions, or ideas. These are highly ethical, even altruistic, requirements and are, not surprisingly, often tested in reality by competition for the three baser, but human, motivating Rs of research: resources, recognition, and reward. Thus, the proper functioning of peer review requires people with detailed knowledge in the area, acquired by or due to similar pursuits and interests, to evaluate—in a fair and unprejudiced way—the proposals and papers of individuals who are competitors for the same dollars (and research goals and objectives) and not to profit intellectually from what they learn in the process. Cast in this light, it is really quite remarkable that the process works at all and is, in fact, generally endorsed, at least in principle, by the scientific community as, by far, the best mechanism for evaluating proposals and reports. It is also not too surprising, however, that the present system is seen by many to be flawed and in need of change. The rather extensive overhaul of peer review by the National Institutes of Health that is a continuing process (Marshall 1997) is a cogent indicator that these concerns are valid.

Several reasons are often put forth to explain why peer review problems appear to be becoming more acute. Invariably, inadequate resources—that is, insufficient funds to pay all the worthy grants—tops the list. Although there was a time when the NIH actually paid essentially all approved grants, there has been a consensus for some time that only about a third of all submissions fit into this worthy category. This is certainly an arguable number, but as long as it is higher than the amount of dollars to cover it, that is of minor importance. This discrepancy then forces review groups, so it is argued, to make difficult choices (and, inevitably, prevents promising research from being done). In effect, this process has been the basis of the successful lobbying of Congress for the past few years, which has achieved real increases in the NIH budget (even though the gap in what is funded and what should be has still not been closed).

Indeed, there is truth in these concerns, but the argument is also a convenient way of glossing over issues that lead to poor, even abusive, peer review practices. Some of this problem is structural, and some is inherent in the competitive nature of research. The latter is clearly a two-edged sword. Competition is, to many, the driving force that sparks originality and creativity. But this force also has a dark side that has become all too visible in the misconduct problems that have been plaguing science, particularly in the United States, for the past ten years. With the exception of sociopaths, most cases of true misconduct—involving falsification, fabrication, or plagiarism—can be directly attributed to situations resulting from the inappropriate desire to achieve status and reward. We cannot seriously expect scientific misconduct to go away when we place such a high premium on awards and other forms of national and international recognition, which, in turn, depend directly on adequate and dependable sources of research funding. Thus, one of the most important qualities necessary for success in research is also a primary factor in impairing its development.

The Career Time Line

To understand peer review of research grants fully, one needs first to comprehend the time line of the career of a typical academic bioscien-

29

tist. While interest in science often begins at an early age (and needs to be cultivated during that time), formal training starts at the undergraduate level and matures during postgraduate training, usually at the predoctoral level. Postdoctoral work completes phase one. Phase two is marked by entry into an independent position, which generally requires competing for research funds. Although variable, this period lasts for about six–seven years and usually culminates in tenure (or the lack thereof). If this phase is successfully accomplished, the individual is now an established researcher and enters the third part of the career, which is more variable in length and is often distinguished with accumulated honors, responsibilities, and the associated recognition. The last and final phase is that of the senior investigator. This is ordinarily the last ten to fifteen years of one's career. For scientists who have not fled to the halls of administration or the front offices of major companies, it is commonly characterized by a slowing in research activities, as manifested in smaller research teams and fewer papers. These, however, are often still innovative and of high quality since they are built on a deep base of experience. This group collectively, scientists in all four stages of their careers, derive their fellowship and research support, for the most part, from government funding.

Although it may seem a little strange, at first, to the uninitiated, the mechanisms for distributing research grants have not basically differed for investigators in the last three phases of their careers (except at the beginning of phase two). This process, which depends critically on review by scientists themselves, treats all investigator-initiated proposals (so-called R01s) competitively; that is, they are reviewed by a study section composed on the basis of expertise (with some balance defined by gender and race but not age). Thus, a young investigator must compete with individuals at the height of their careers and with senior scientists, maybe not as active but with twenty-five–thirty years' experience. The rationale for this system has its roots in the belief that we should support the best (most competitive) science and that this is not defined by age. The realization, however, that some differences were directly related to age did eventually lead to the development of a new NIH grant category, the FIRST award, which gave smaller amounts of money for three years to help young investigators when it became clear that they were having trouble competing for the diminishing resources. Interestingly, but perhaps predictably, the NIH is now considering extending these to five years and increasing the amounts of money so that these young researchers are not impaired exactly at the time when they should have the maximum freedom to make their mark (Wadman 1979). In effect, there is movement toward separating the R01 pool on an age basis.

There are, in fact, compelling reasons to look at the other end of the grantee spectrum as well. Study sections are generally composed of scientists in the third part of their careers (but often skewed toward the early part of it). If, as would normally be expected, one applies one's own experiences and standards to the evaluations at hand, there would be no basis to evaluate the proposal of a more senior investigator, where their greater experience might suggest a more risky but potentially more rewarding approach to a problem. The recently promulgated changes in evaluation criteria (Marshall 1979), which emphasize five categories and include, notably and correctly, innovation as well as a consideration of the investigator's credentials, seem to recognize the importance of such approaches rather than the mundane and tiresome emphasis on practicality (usually in the form of preliminary data) that seems more and more to be a euphemism for a situation in which the proposed experiments have already been done. In an atmosphere of competition (for those very same dollars), and with a little king-of-the-hill mentality among the younger, more aggressive (and arrogant) members of a review group, however, a failure to appreciate innovative ideas (which are not as easy to recognize as one might think) and an unwillingness to accept that experience and judgment may be as good (or even better) predictors of what might work, may dull the enthusiasm of a review group for a proposal, with a resulting catastrophic effect on the priority score. The relatively recent practice of placing a few senior scientists on established panels is clearly an admission of this problem. Some grant categories for senior investigators, although limited in scope, do address this concern as well, but they are hardly widespread or equitably distributed.

A Simple Reorganization

In a perfect world, grants would be reviewed anonymously, and only the science (and not the investigator or the institution) would be considered. Unfortunately, this is not practical since experts in the field would recognize the investigator (unless new) either through the description of the proposed research or, more likely, from the summary of past progress. Sadly, even this situation would not alter the basic imbalances inherently introduced by age and experience.

What is really needed is a simple reorganization that would deal effectively with this and would divide proposals into categories that generally correspond to the three phases of academic careers and have them reviewed by panels composed predominantly of scientists at corresponding levels—in a word, put the *peer* back into peer review. The appropriate distribution of funds to pay these categories would ensure that all levels of investigators remained viable and that competition was at least on a level playing field. There is an assumption here that each category (or career-phase group) brings something different to the research enterprise and therefore should be retained. A second, also simple, change is to remove all financial and budgetary data from the initial review. Finally, the amounts of money for each category should have a ceiling, with the largest awards going to the middle group. Older (or younger) scientists could have the option to be considered in the more competitive group if they felt so inclined. Importantly, these changes do not eliminate competition, but they do alter the emphasis so that the effect is more likely to be positive than now.

Bias in reviewing will not be easily eliminated. It is not limited to age: nepotism and sexism are examples of other problem areas (Wenneras and Wold 1997). Although structural changes will help, alterations in the way both the lay and scientific communities view reward and recognition of scientific accomplishment will certainly be a perquisite for material improvement. Any change that improves peer review, however, would certainly have the effect of boosting morale in the scientific community and increasing productivity without adding a single dime to the federal research budget. Scientists could also make a much more compelling case for their appeals for increased support if they spent a little time on improving their part of the research enterprise.

References

E. Marshall. 1997. *Science* 276:888–89.
M. Wadman. 1997. *Nature* 387:834.
C. Wenneras and Wold, A. 1997. *Nature* 387:341–43.

PART TWO

The Case for Public Support
of Biomedical Research

6

Support for Basic Biomedical Research: How Scientific Breakthroughs Occur

Arthur Kornberg

From 1942 to 1952, after my medical training, I was at the NIH where I was introduced to full-time research. I regard NIH, as do so many others, as my true alma mater. At the NIH, I was also involved in the early development of the extramural grants program and have depended on its grant entirely for the past forty-five years that I have spent in the medical schools of Washington University in St. Louis and at Stanford. For about as many years I have been concerned about the support of basic biomedical research—that it be long term, that it nourish training and talent, and that it rely on creativity from the bottom up rather than on strategic objectives imposed from the top down.

In reflecting on the history of biomedical science in this century, I often resort to a hunting metaphor. The microbe hunters in the early decades discovered the microbial sources of the major scourges: tuberculosis, plague, cholera. They were followed by the vitamin hunters, who discovered that other scourges—scurvy, rickets, beriberi—were caused by the lack of a dietary substance, named vitamins. In the fifth and sixth decades, the enzyme hunters occupied the stage, explaining how the enzyme machinery depends on vitamins to make cells grow and function. Now they have been eclipsed by the gene hunters, the genetic engineers who use recombinant DNA technology to identify and clone genes, the blueprints for the enzymes, and introduce them into bacteria and plants to create factories for the massive production of hormones and vaccines for medicine and better crops for agriculture. Biotechnology has become a multibillion dollar industry.

Almost daily we see newspaper reports of discoveries by gene hunters of a defective gene responsible for one or another disease, as well as genes for predisposition to cancer and other illnesses. In view of the inexorable progress in science, we can expect that the gene hunters will be replaced in the spotlight. I have wondered whether the truly novel hunters will be those who apply the techniques of the enzyme and gene hunters to the functions of the brain. What to call them? The head hunters.

During this twentieth century, with its succession of hunters and golden ages in medical science, the current age of gene hunting is undeniably the most golden. We have an inexhaustible supply of genes and simple and efficient techniques to track and capture them. Genetic engineering and related biotechnologies represent the most revolutionary advance in the history of biological and medical science. The term *revolutionary* is generally overused, but not here. The effects of this advance on medicine, agriculture, and industry have not been exaggerated.

Yet even more revolutionary but generally unnoticed, even by scientists, is a development that lacks a name or obvious applications but will lead to even more remarkable and unanticipated practical applications. I refer to the coalescence of the numerous basic biological and medical sciences into a single, unified discipline, which has emerged because it is expressed in a single universal language, the language of chemistry.

Much of life can be understood in rational terms if expressed in the language of chemistry. It is an international language, a language without dialects, a language for all of time, and a language that explains where we came from, what we are, and where the physical world will allow us to go. Chemical language has great aesthetic beauty and links the physical sciences to the biological sciences.

Yet, when I entered medical school in 1937, the importance of chemistry was hardly noticed. It was also a serious question whether the genes, then an abstraction, operated by known physical principles. Of course, we now understand and examine genetics and heredity in simple chemical terms as DNA. DNA in the chromosomes and genes is easily analyzed, synthesized, and rearranged. Species are modified at will. It is no longer a question of whether we can sequence the 3 billion units of the human genome, but rather when it will be completed.

In science today, we possess phenomenal capacities to acquire and integrate unprecedented quantities of sophisticated data. Yet, in this time of informational plenty, we are beset by serious problems that threaten our scientific enterprise. For this occasion, I have selected just two among the many that warrant our concern, whether we be scientists or lay people.

I want to consider the antiscience attitudes and scientific illiteracy in society and the lack of support for basic science. The first problem is the rising tide of public fear, distrust, and rejection of science, both chemical and biological.

Chemistry has had a poor image for some time. The DuPont slogan: "Better things for better living . . . through chemistry" is now simply: "Better things for better living." No chemistry. The merger of the Chase Manhattan and the even larger Chemical Bank resulted only in the Chase Manhattan; no "chemical" in its name. In fact, the only times we hear something good said of chemistry these days are references, as in newspaper articles, to the good chemistry of the Green Bay Packers or the improved chemistry between the president and Congress.

The image of biologists has not been doing well either. Hollywood, lacking Communists for culprits and squeamish about racial bashing, has used doctors and scientists as their villains in recent years. Perhaps Hollywood has taken its cue from news reports that science is wracked with fraud. People fail to recognize that the practice of science defines rather strict boundaries for behavior that are effective in all but the rare instance, one in a thousand or less, of the irrational and the criminal. In the practice of science, the more startling the claim, the more it attracts attention, and if false, the sooner it is exposed.

This brings me to the second problem, the lack of adequate financial support for science, a poverty worsened by severe pressures to engage in targeted research such as the treatment of breast cancer and AIDS or the development of medical technologies to improve the economy.

I am reminded of the story of the surgeon who, while jogging around a lake, spotted a man drowning. He dove in, dragged the victim ashore, and resuscitated him. He resumed his jogging, only to see two more drownings. He also saw a colleague, a professor of biochemistry nearby, witnessing the scene, absorbed in thought. He called to him to go after one while he went after the other. When the biochemist was slow to respond, he shouted, "Why aren't you doing something?" The biochemist said, "I am doing something. I'm desperately trying to figure out who's throwing all these people in the lake."

This parable is not intended to convey a lack of regard for fundamental issues among clinicians or a callousness among scientists.

37

Rather, it portrays the reality that a serious problem, a war on disease, must be fought on several fronts. Some contribute their special skills to the distressed individual while others try to gain the broad knowledge base necessary to cope with present and future enemies.

Five years ago, Bernadine Healy, then director of the NIH, developed a strategic plan for medical research. Such plans are fundamentally flawed because discoveries are commonly serendipitous. The best plan over many decades has been no plan. For lack of essential knowledge, timetables for assaults on particular disease targets have had little meaning. Nor could we have anticipated the confrontations with novel diseases, such as AIDS, Legionnaires' disease, septic shock, and drug-resistant tuberculosis.

Medical research is still more a game of pool than billiards. You score points regardless of which pocket the ball goes into. This was eloquently explained by Harold Varmus, the present director of NIH, in addressing the "Conference to Establish a National Plan on Breast Cancer." He made it clear that a specific disease model is far too narrow a target to encompass the huge complexities of a disease process, such as cancer or AIDS.

A well-designed plan, by its nature, cannot lay the groundwork for the utterly novel techniques that make possible major transformations in the acquisition and application of knowledge. The success of the NIH that has changed the face of medicine in the post–World War II period was not planned. This extraordinary success is owed to channeling a major fraction of the budgets of the Heart, Cancer, and twenty other disease institutes to noncategorical, basic research. Had this money been spent instead in palliating these various diseases, the current advances in preventing and curing them would have been squandered. How tragic that the NIH, with a budget for basic research of only 1 percent of the health care dollar and the best investment for improving the quality of medicine, is faced each year with arbitrary and devastating cuts for research and training.

The breakthrough of recombinant DNA and genetic engineering was based on the discoveries of enzymes that make, break, and seal DNA. All these basic advances were made in academic laboratories built and supported almost entirely by funds from the NIH. For thirty years, my research on the biosynthesis of the building blocks of nucleic acids, their assembly in DNA replication, and the training of over a hundred young scientists, was funded with many millions of dollars without any promise or expectation that this research would lead to marketable products or procedures. No industrial organization had, or would ever have, the resources or disposition to invest in such long-range, apparently impractical programs. We carried out these studies to satisfy our curiosity. Yet, to my great pleasure, such studies of the replication, repair, and rearrangements of DNA have had many practical benefits.

They provided the reagents that made recombinant DNA and genetic engineering possible. By defining the pathways of assembling DNA from its building blocks, we provided the basis for the design of most drugs used today in the chemotherapy of cancer and the treatment of autoimmune diseases, AIDS, and herpes. This knowledge is essential to understanding the repair of DNA, so important in the aging process, and for understanding mutations and the origin of cancers and aging.

It may seem unreasonable and impractical, call it counterintuitive, even to scientists, to solve an urgent problem, such as a disease, by pursuing apparently unrelated questions in basic biology or chemistry. Yet, the pursuit of curiosity about the basic facts of nature has proved throughout the history of medical science to be the most practical, the most cost-effective route to successful drugs and devices.

Investigations that seemed totally irrelevant to any practical objective have yielded most of the major discoveries of medicine: X-rays were discovered by a physicist observing discharges in vacuum tubes; penicillin came from enzyme studies of bacterial lysis; and the polio vaccine, from learning how to grow cells in culture. Cisplatin, a widely used drug in cancer chemotherapy, was a fortuitous discovery in studies of how electric fields affect the growth of bacteria. As mentioned, genetic engineering and recombinant DNA depended on reagents developed in exploring DNA biochemistry. All these discoveries have come from the pursuit of curiosity about questions in physics, chemistry, and biology, apparently unrelated at the outset to a specific medical or practical problem.

A few years ago, at a meeting in Washington celebrating the bicentennial of the U.S. Patent Office, a remarkable truth emerged. It was agreed that the age-old aphorism "Necessity is the mother of invention" is usually wrong. Generally, the reverse proved to be true: Invention is the mother of necessity. Inventions only later become necessities.

Time and again, inventors created things that had to wait many years to be recognized for their practical value. Nobody needed the airplane, the FM radio, television, or the quantum mechanics that led to lasers. The transistor created in the Bell Labs in 1947 was only a curiosity to its inventors and received scant attention when unveiled to the public. Take xerography. It took Chester Carlson, the inventor of the Xerox process, six years to interest a company in his invention and twenty years before the first commercial copier was produced. Fax machines were invented thirty years ago, but it took a deteriorated postal service among other factors to make them the necessities they are today.

Quite clearly, even industrial inventions emerge from a creative process. As such, they are haphazard rather than goal-oriented. The process of invention conflicts with prudent business strategy. A pioneering invention, almost by definition, is profoundly different from what a company has been doing. It is commercially unproved and therefore riskier than the established business.

The lessons to be learned from this history should be crystal clear. It is crucial for a society, a culture, a company, a medical school to understand the nature of the creative process and to provide for its support. No matter how counterintuitive it may seem, basic research is the lifeline of practical advances in medicine; pioneering inventions are the source of industrial strength.

The future is invented, not predicted. Great innovations, whether in art, literature, or science, seldom take the world by storm. They must be cultivated to be understood, understood before they can be properly appreciated.

Of course, it is important that basic discoveries be promptly and wisely applied to solve practical problems. They are. The recent applications of biotechnology to medicine have given us major insights into diabetes, cancer, and other metabolic diseases. Will these approaches and techniques be equally effective when applied to the human brain and behavior? Over the long term, they will.

The overriding issue in biomedical science is how to give our abundant scientific talent the resources to exploit the extraordinary new technologies to advance knowledge. Currently, a pervasive mood among productive biomedical scientists makes them fear for continued grant support, persuades them to choose safe and practical projects over the untried and adventurous, and tempts their interest in commercial ventures. This state clearly discourages young people from entering science and drives others to abandon science for business, law, and medical practice.

Scientists are beseeched to make the case for support of biomedical research with their fellow citizens, to be friend-raisers in the community, and to persuade their congressmen to increase the NIH budget. Then they are berated for doing none of these things. Their friends in the community and in the Congress fail to realize that scientists, as a group, are self-selected for their interest in molecules and cells and their disinterest in people and politics. Unlike virtually every other segment of society—doctors, lawyers, businessmen, farmers— they fail individually and collectively to lobby for their cause.

40

The most prestigious of our scientific societies, the National Academy of Sciences, through its National Research Council, makes awesome contributions of factual information from highway construction to child care. Yet, as a matter of policy, it has refrained from efforts to maintain, let alone increase, federal support for basic research. As a private organization with quasi-governmental status, the academy has been fearful of appearing political. As for the lobbying efforts of the major scientific societies, they, by their own admission and despite occasional heroic interventions, have been amateurish and grossly inadequate. Valiant pleadings by Research!America; the cancer, heart, and fifty other disease societies; universities and medical schools; and concerned individuals are heard as splintered, divisive, incoherent, and unfocused constituencies and fail to inform our administrators and legislators of the value of basic biomedical research.

For its long-term support, we need to convey this message, "If you think research is expensive, try disease." We need to inform our fellow citizens, especially at this time of severe budgetary restraints and in competition with imperative and urgent social programs, that throughout the history of medical science, the major advances in diagnosis and the prevention of and treatment of disease were based on the curiosity of biologists, chemists, and physicists unrelated to the ultimate application of this basic knowledge to the development of vaccines, drugs, and devices.

I see nothing wrong, base, or narrow in organizing and operating a national organization of scientists to promote health science. With proper leadership, such an organization could enroll a sufficient number of dues-paying bioscience investigators and with contributions from medical schools, pharmaceutical companies, and private donors could maintain an annual budget of $3–5 million, enough to support a staff of twenty or so people skilled in attracting attention and informing the public. The scientists in every one of the 435 congressional districts would respond eagerly to requests to present their research and its significance to lay groups in their communities. So, for once, scientists would be seen actively promoting science for the public welfare and relieved of being criticized for indifference and selfishness. And Congress and the people would be grateful to hear one sustained, reasoned voice making the case for biomedical research support rather than the babble of an undisciplined chorus.

7

The Economists' Case for Biomedical Research

Lynne G. Zucker and Michael R. Darby

The world . . . is only beginning to see that the wealth of a nation consists more than anything else in the number of superior men that it harbors. . . . Geniuses are ferments; and when they come together, as they have done in certain lands at certain times, the whole population seems to share in the higher energy which they awaken. The effects are incalculable and often not easy to trace in detail, but they are pervasive and momentous.

WILLIAM JAMES

The time has long passed when history was seen as the biographies of great men—and occasionally great women. The very idea smacks of elitism and conflicts with our ideas of communalism and teamwork. Nonetheless, our research on the development of the science underlying biotechnology and its commercial applications has led us to conclude that, at least during the period of ferment following a breakthrough change in science, particular great men and women play crucial roles in the development and diffusion of the science and in the formation and transformation of the industries that apply it.

According to our findings, the scientists most productive in academic publications also play a significant role in determining where and when firms enter biotechnology and which of them are most successful. We also found that the productivity of those scientists is en-

See note at end of chapter for acknowledgments.

hanced during their period of commercial involvement. To the extent that they are involved in the commercialization of their discoveries, these (primarily academic) scientist-entrepreneurs are thus able to pursue their scientific and financial goals simultaneously, indeed symbiotically. Before we turn to the evidence that led us to these conclusions, it is appropriate to put this research in a broader context.

Government Support of Basic Research

Governmental support for basic research is motivated primarily not by direct commercial gains that the discovering scientists and their employers can capture—although those rewards may be important considerations for the private participants in basic research—but by the belief that the most important gains cannot or should not be captured by the inventors through intellectual property rights or otherwise. The *cannot* arises because some externalities or "spillovers" are inevitable in which basic science discoveries lead to a host of further advances, some of which may have commercial import but none of which can be specifically traced to and made to pay royalties as the fruit of one or more basic science discoveries. Other benefits of basic science discoveries may have no commercial value but be of substantial social value in making us better able to understand and cope with the universe in which we live, whether as individuals or collectively through our government.

The *should not* arises because basic scientific discoveries frequently have such wide-ranging implications—both with respect to the field of application and to the time since their discovery—that if other scientists and inventors were deterred from using a discovery because of a high cost of or refusal to license by the discoverer considerable social loss could occur. To some extent this *should not* is incorporated in our patent law, which denies patent rights to discoverers of basic laws of nature or mathematical formulas, regardless of their novelty, nonobviousness, and commercial utility. Traditional academic norms of openness and free publication also embody the principle that basic discoveries are properly placed in the public domain.

Public policy in the 1980s—particularly in the Bayh-Dole Act and subsequent executive orders—has turned away somewhat from the view that basic discoveries supported in whole or part by public funds should be dedicated to the public domain. Sad experience has shown that particularly where scientific innovations need substantial further development or marketing expenditures to yield commercial products, they have lain fallow since no firm has the incentive, for example, to prove a potentially life-saving drug's safety and effectiveness if generic producers can free-ride on that investment. Thus, the classic tension between static efficiency (free use of basic ideas) and dynamic efficiency (incentives for inventive activity through patents) is incomplete in cases where common ownership of an idea eliminates the incentive to invest in developing commercial applications. Of course, the expected value of these patent rights to the scientists and their employers is reflected in lower costs to the government for any given level of basic research, and large externalities still remain.

If basic science yields social benefits far in excess of any private returns—and those private returns are reduced by practical, legal, and ethical limits—then it makes sense for government and private eleemosynary institutions to support that important activity. A difficult problem for policy makers—which we cannot solve here—is how much support is the right amount and how to allocate that support to the most productive researchers. Our research indicates that a small number of extraordinarily talented scientists play a crucial role in total scientific productivity, but one should not conclude that support can be limited to only this core group. First, the star scientists are able to achieve much more as leaders of a larger scientific enterprise, including not only scientists who work directly on their team but also others who fill in the details of their breakthroughs. Furthermore, we would have far fewer star scientists as well as their collaborators if an attractive research career were available only for those few who turn out to be rarely gifted. Finally, it is difficult to identify some of the most creative scientists until they have proved the possibility of what was believed impossible.

For these reasons, our nation has supported basic research across a broad range of science. That support reflects the reality that it is impossible to predict which field will next experience a breakthrough invention with important social and economic benefits. The early years of scientific revolutions are essentially come-as-you-are affairs, and nations that do not have the research teams that either make the discoveries or quickly build on them are unlikely to play an important role in any consequent formation or transformation of industries as scientific breakthroughs are transferred to technology.

The arguments for governmental support for basic research in general apply with particular force to biomedical research. Patent protection is less fully available, and the market cannot be expected in any case to value that portion of savings in medical costs and lost income that accrue to the government. Government and private charitable institutions have emphasized support of biomedical research for decades. Nonetheless, in 1970 biology was not seen as a cutting-edge science, nor was basic research in biology expected to be a leading source of medical breakthroughs. Although support was adequate, no national science and technology policy focused on pushing biology as a source of medical or other technology. The revolution in the science begun in 1973 and its fast application as biotechnology changed that landscape drastically, and funding grew rapidly with the science's ability to use it productively.

Development and Commercialization of Bioscience

This chapter examines the process of growth and commercial application as an interesting and useful subject of scientific inquiry. Our purposes are not normative in the sense of prescribing what should be done from an ethical, policy, or management point of view but rather to understand the process and how it works. As with basic research in bioscience, the applications must follow that fundamental understanding.

Although grounded in extensive fieldwork and case studies, our research is primarily quantitative, and the foundation of our methodology is the operational definition of a set of highly productive scientists whom we term *star scientists* or simply *stars*. The primary criterion for selection as a star was the discovery of more than forty genetic sequences as reported in GenBank (1990) through April 1990.[1] Twenty-two scientists, however, were included based on writing twenty or more articles, each reporting one or more genetic sequence discoveries.[2] In the 1990s, sequence discovery has become routinized and is no longer such a useful measure of research success. These 327 stars were only three-fourths of 1 percent of the authors in GenBank (1990) but accounted for 17.3 percent of the published articles, almost twenty-two times as many articles as the average scientist. Clearly, focusing on genetic sequences means that we have missed some great scientists working in less prominent areas of biotechnology such as monoclonal antibodies and that we have included some scientists who, while hard working, may lack the genius and vision that we believe are so important around the time of a Kuhnian revolution in which the standard ways of doing things are being replaced. Nonetheless, just as enriching

---

1. GenBank has the advantage of containing a complete census of genetic sequence discoveries regardless of language or location of the discovering scientist or journal of publication.

2. Scientists advised that some sequence discoveries are more difficult than others and thus merit an article reporting only one sequence. Therefore, we included scientists with twenty or more discovery articles to avoid excluding scientists who specialized in more difficult problems.

45

uranium increases only the proportion of U-238 to U-235 to obtain a fissionable level, our procedure does not have to be a perfect screen to be usable for empirical analysis.

Our 327 stars were listed as authors on 4,061 distinct articles in major journals. These articles were hand collected and used to identify and locate institutional affiliations at the time of publication for each of our stars and their coauthors who were either other stars or "collaborators" (6,082 scientists worldwide). Of these scientists, 207 stars and 4,004 collaborators published in the United States up to 1990.[3]

Using a variety of commercial data bases and directories as well as an early proprietary source, we have compiled a firm data set including 751 distinct U.S. firms for which we could determine a zip code and a date of initial use of biotechnology. Of these 751 firms, 511 were entrants, 150 incumbents, and 90 (including 18 joint ventures) could not be definitively classified. By 1990, 52 of the 751 firms had ceased to exist or merged into other firms.

In addition to the original GenBank (our star-collaborative-article-affiliation data and firm data sets), we have compiled data bases on local economic conditions for each of America's 183 functional economic areas (hereafter "regions") identified by the U.S. Bureau of Economic Analysis, the U.S. universities granting doctoral degrees in the relevant fields, and other significant information.

These rich data sets have permitted us to identify some effects that are "often not easy to trace in detail," but, which seem to us (as they did to William James), "pervasive and momentous." We shall now present an overview of results primarily from the United States that illustrate the crucial and symbiotic roles of the star scientists in both science and industry. The next section presents an analysis of the diffusion process around and following the 1973 breakthrough discovery of Stanley Cohen and Herbert Boyer. The section "The Formation and Transformation of Industry" reports on the determinants of where and when firms began using the new biotechnology. "Star Scientists and the Success of Biotechnology Firms" establishes what makes these firms more or less successful in actually using the technology commercially in the United States. Whether commercial involvement helps or hurts the scientific productivity of star scientists based on both U.S. and worldwide data is addressed in "Commercial Involvement and the Scientific Productivity of Star Scientists." In "National Innovation Systems That Promote Stars' Commercial Involvement," the expe-

---

3. We have recently completed extending the set of articles to 1993, but the analyses reported in this chapter are confined to the original data set unless explicitly stated otherwise.

rience of the Asia-Pacific Economic Cooperation countries in biotechnology is contrasted with that of Europe. We conclude with a brief summary of what we have learned so far and the questions that we yet hope to answer.

The Diffusion of Tacit Knowledge

The key scientific breakthrough in bioscience was the 1973 discovery by Stanford professor Stanley Cohen and University of California–San Francisco professor Herbert Boyer of the basic technique for recombinant DNA (reported in Cohen, Chang, Boyer, and Helling 1973). Today, biotechnology refers principally to the application of genetic engineering based on taking a gene from one organism and implanting it in another and production of the outcome of this process.[4] The selection of promising lines and the gene transfer itself require very special skills and talents, which were quite rare at least until the early 1980s, although the production part of biotechnology has been more accessible.

Star scientists are outliers in the distribution of productivity in a breakthrough area of bioscience. By virtue of the discoveries that these stars have made, they have "intellectual human capital" that other scientists value highly. The typical model of knowledge diffusion assumes that these other scientists can easily replicate the discoveries by talking to the discovering scientists or reading their publications. Thus, after a discovery is made, it is assumed that as quickly as the new knowledge reaches other scientists, they can immediately build on it. That is, knowledge rapidly becomes disembodied from its discoverer and can be transmitted as information through discussion and publication.

Natural Excludability. We argue instead that scientific discoveries vary in the degree to which others can be excluded from making use of them (Zucker, Darby, and Brewer 1994, 1997). Inherent in the discovery itself is its degree of *natural excludability*: information about many new discoveries, especially an "invention of a method of inventing" (Griliches 1957), is so costly to transfer because of either its complexity or its tacitness that others are effectively excluded (see Nelson 1959; Arrow 1962, 1974; Nelson and Winter 1982; Rosenberg 1982). At the

---

4. The other basic technology is cell fusion (also termed monoclonal antibodies, MABs, or hybridomas) in which lymphocytes are fused with myeloma cells to create rapidly proliferating antibody-producing cells (see Sindelar 1992 and 1993 for more detail).

extreme, scientists wishing to build on the new knowledge must first acquire hands-on experience.[5] If scientists cannot gain access to a research team or laboratory setting with that know-how, then working in the new area may be very difficult, if not impossible.

One indicator of the high degree of natural excludability is the difficulties encountered in making the "enabling disclosure" required for a valid U.S. patent application—a disclosure that will enable the public to practice the innovation once the patent expires. Because of the inherent difficulty in disclosing the art used to obtain the invention so that it can be readily replicated, patents are now obtainable by biotech inventors who disclose their invention by placing a culture in a recognized public depository. (See Eisenberg 1987 for a discussion of the related litigation and legislation.) Natural excludability was so high that a new method of disclosure—"disclosure by deposit"—had to be invented.

Copublication. A second measure of the degree of natural excludability is the extent to which scientists who have not worked in the genetic sequence area before can enter on their own or need to learn from doing bench-level science with a more experienced investigator. To quantify these largely invisible working relationships, we use a copublishing measure we developed elsewhere to provide a novel analysis of the diffusion of scientific knowledge: we measure scientific collaboration as those who publish together and then collect related data on characteristics of the scientific research team.[6] We track each

---

5. In principle, even if tacit knowledge is important, it can be obtained by reverse engineering, but the cost of this approach may be prohibitive relative to working with an experienced practitioner.

6. We build here on a novel empirical measure we developed in earlier research: "copublishing," examining all scientists who publish together, to measure who the stars are working with at the bench-science level and which organizations are involved in the collaboration (by obtaining the organizational affiliation of all scientists). We have previously used our measure to examine reciprocal productivity effects of star scientists working with scientists in firms (see our discussion of these results in "Star Scientists and the Success of Biotechnology Firms," below), effects of organizational boundaries as information envelopes slowing diffusion of scientific knowledge, and size and geography of scientific networks used by firms (Zucker, Darby, and Armstrong 1994, 1997a; Zucker and Darby 1996; Zucker, Darby, Brewer, and Peng 1996; Liebeskind, Oliver, Zucker, and Brewer 1996; and Zucker, Brewer, Oliver, and Liebeskind 1993). The validity of our copublishing indicator for the existence of contractual or ownership relationships with firms has been confirmed through extensive interviews with university scientists and administrators, and with firm scientists, CEOs, and corporate board members (for U.S. exam-

scientist who has ever published an article reporting a genetic sequence discovery listed in GenBank (1994): in all, 84,461 individual authors entered GenBank from 1969 through 1993, joining a handful of pioneers who managed to report sequence discoveries before 1969. Together they published 66,070 articles—we exclude only unpublished sources and patents because the information is often incomplete.

We operationalize a measure of natural excludability by distinguishing between "new" authors (those who have never published before in GenBank) and "old" authors (those whose publications have appeared previously in GenBank). Initially, by definition, the first scientific collaboration to write an article reporting a genetic-sequence discovery must have all new authors as defined here. After that initial discovery, however, there are authors who have published on the discovery before. The extent to which initial publication by scientists new to GenBank involves a bench-level working relationship with at least one other scientist who demonstrably knows the techniques already, indicates the degree of natural excludability after the breakthrough discovery is made. That category would include anyone who has already published at least once in GenBank. Obviously, bench-level transfers of tacit scientific knowledge do not necessarily result in copublication. A student, for example, might learn the technique as a research assistant without earning coauthorship or might publish a dissertation solo, even where the chairman of the dissertation committee might in other circumstances share in authorship credit. If new authors predominantly copublish with old authors, however, the case is strong for a significant degree of natural excludability.

If most new scientists are publishing with at least one old author, natural excludability would appear to be high; if most new entrants to GenBank can do the research either by himself or herself or with all new authors, natural excludability would appear to be low. Breakthrough discoveries seldom result in only one type of copublishing, so the issue is the balance between the two. As we can see in figure 7–1, new authors enter GenBank predominantly by publishing with old authors, with this mode accounting for 81 percent of entry from 1969 through 1992.[7] Excluding sole-authored articles, which may be dissertations for new authors and review articles by established au-

---

ples, see Zucker and Darby 1995; Zucker, Brewer, Oliver, and Liebeskind 1993).

7. Reports of publications for 1993 were incomplete in February 1994, so that year has been excluded from the figure and these calculations. In the incomplete reports for 1993, entry with old authors amounted to 83 percent of total entry.

FIGURE 7–1
New Authors in GenBank by Articles Written with
Old Authors, 1969–1992
(number of authors)

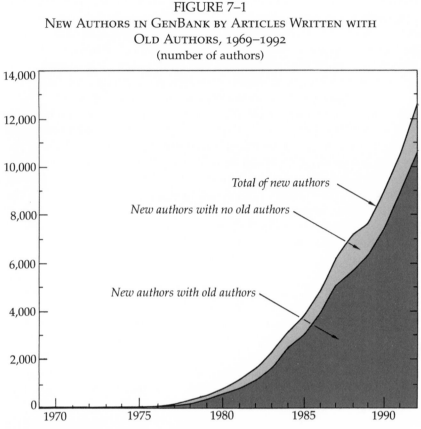

Source: Calculations of the authors based on GenBank (1994).

thors, new authors write exclusively with other new authors 36 percent
less frequently than old authors write exclusively with other old authors.[8]

The high degree of natural excludability inherent in the biotechnology breakthroughs is important for understanding the process of
technology transfer given that the scientific knowledge had high commercial value. High natural excludability explains both why discovering star scientists might be motivated to become involved with

---

8. Sole-authored articles account for only 6.5 percent of the authorships of
new authors and 7.8 percent of the authorships of old authors over this period.
Interestingly, new sole authors become more frequent later in the period, as
the value of the tacit knowledge declined as it became more widespread (see
also Zucker, Darby, Brewer, and Peng 1996).

firms—they have the opportunity to earn extraordinary returns to their intellectual human capital—and why firms might be motivated to work with star scientists—these discovering scientists have very rare tacit knowledge.[9]

The Formation and Transformation of Industry

In Zucker, Darby, and Brewer (1994, 1997), we have examined what determined where and when U.S. firms entered biotechnology in the formative and transformative years of the industries in which it has been applied. In the United States, the bulk of these firms were "entrants" (newly formed to commercialize biotechnology), and the remainder, "incumbents" (adopting the new technology to remain competitive in their existing businesses such as pharmaceuticals), or difficult to classify cases such as joint ventures between entrants and incumbents.

We expected that the probability that a firm would enter on any given day in any given region would depend on both the endowment of intellectual human capital specific to the technology in the region and the general economic conditions of the region. We measured intellectual human capital by the numbers of stars and their collaborators actively publishing in the region and year, the number of universities in the region with a relevant department receiving top-quality ratings in the 1981 National Research Council study of doctoral programs, and the number of faculty with federal support in the region in 1979–1980. General economic conditions were measured by the region's total employment (all industries) and average wages per job and the national S&P 500 earnings-price ratio for the year.

In our cited papers, we have used a variety of appropriate statistical techniques to explore the process of industry formation and transformation. These analyses show that the rate of entry of firms in a region and year is significantly increased by higher numbers of actively publishing stars, top-quality universities, federally supported bioscience researchers, and average wages. The other variables examined do not have stable, statistically significant effects. When entry equations are estimated separately for entrants and incumbents, similar coefficients are obtained, suggesting that incumbents, like new entrants, chose to establish their biotechnology operations where and when the science base was available, not necessarily where their existing research facilities were. These results point to a second factor that,

---

9. The same scientists often have the genius and vision to apply commercially valuable techniques in the most promising areas of research.

in combination with natural excludability, leads to the geographic localization and agglomeration of the related industry: star scientists are not likely to give up their university positions and labs and, because of the value of their time, are also likely to form or collaborate only with firms close to their homes or university offices. Extending our work to Japan, we found qualitatively similar results, although the intellectual human capital variables were significantly weaker relative to the other economic variables in Japan, consistent with differences in geography and institutions (Darby and Zucker 1996).

These results are entirely consistent with the important literature on "geographically localized knowledge spillovers," which rely on geographic proximity to identify the impact of university-based science and engineering innovations on local economic growth (see, for example, Jaffe 1989; Jaffe, Trajtenberg, and Henderson 1993; Acs, Audretsch, and Feldman 1992). Our findings validate the star scientist variable as a measure of the intellectual human capital that varies over time and place, providing highly significant and distinct explanatory power from standard measures of the quality and quantity of university research.[10]

The most notable surprise for the authors was that the number of collaborators, which we took to be a measure of the training function of the university and the specialized labor in the region, was not generally significant, although sometimes entering positively in the latter half of the 1980s when separate coefficients were estimated by time period. This finding suggests that the effect on entry is related more directly to the research activities of the star scientists than to the number of students who want to live and work in firms near their alma maters and thesis advisers. To shed more light on the role of star scientists, we switched our unit of analysis to individual firms and their relationship with particular stars.

Star Scientists and the Success of Biotechnology Firms

Zucker, Darby, and Armstrong (1994, 1997a) examined what determines which California firms using biotechnology are most successful. Work underway for the United States as a whole (Zucker, Darby, and Armstrong 1997b) and Japan confirms that qualitatively similar state-

---

10. We suspect that more or better screens would identify top scientists in other aspects of modern biotechnology, which are not captured by genetic sequence discoveries, and would reduce or even eliminate the separate significance of top-quality universities and federally supported university researchers.

ments can be made for those larger samples, but here we will confine our discussion to the peer-reviewed results for California.

The first question was what to use for a measure of success. Financial returns or capitalization would eliminate from the sample many firms that are not publicly owned and firms that use biotechnology within a relatively small subunit. We adopted the strategy of explaining counts of products and employment growth after 1989 by variables describing each firm and the region in which it operates up to 1989.

Because of the long time (up to ten years) for testing and approval by the Federal Drug Administration of pharmaceutical products, we examined counts of both products in development and on the market as of 1991. Many of the most valuable products were still in development, while the number on the market was a noisy measure because some firms sell numerous relatively low-value reagents. Employment growth is not a perfect measure of success either, but in biotechnology it serves well to separate the firms that are flourishing, going nowhere, or shrinking.[11]

The explanatory variables used in these regressions were counts of articles written by stars affiliated with the firm, by ("linked") local academic stars as coauthors with firm scientists, and by other ("untied") academic stars in the region who are neither affiliated nor linked to the firm on the article; a dummy variable indicating whether the firm is a new entrant (born after 1975); the elapsed time up to 1989 since the firm's entry into biotechnology; and a second dummy variable indicating whether the firm uses the recombinant DNA technology. Table 7–1 displays key regressions reported in Zucker, Darby, and Armstrong (1997a).

The one variable with a significantly positive effect on all measures of firm success is the number of articles by linked stars, the local academic scientist-entrepreneurs who often possess a significant equity or founding interest in the firm. These coefficients are interpreted graphically in figure 7–2, which shows the expected number of products in development and on the market, as well as employment growth, for firms with average values of the other variables and, alternatively, zero, two, or five articles written by firm scientists with an academic star. Just two such linked articles results in about one more

---

11. Because of the nature of the data, it was appropriate to estimate the product-count variables by Poisson regressions and the employment-growth equation by a modified two-stage Heckman procedure to correct for selectivity or response bias for firms reporting no change. The modified two-stage Heckman procedure was econometrically appropriate but resulted in no real improvement over the more familiar ordinary least squares estimates.

TABLE 7–1

REGRESSIONS EXPLAINING THE SUCCESS OF BIOTECH FIRMS
IN CALIFORNIA

Variables	Coefficients (standard errors)		
	Products in development[a]	Products on the market[a]	Employment growth[b]
Constant	−1.9324‡	1.4953‡	51.022
	(0.2796)	(0.1085)	(252.53)
Count of articles by	0.0001	−0.0006‡	−0.7130
stars untied to firm	(0.0003)	(0.0002)	(0.4256)
Count of articles by	0.3197‡	0.1143‡	172.17†
firm-linked stars	(0.0161)	(0.0140)	(78.157)
Count of articles by	0.0006	0.0024‡	−4.3847
firm-affiliated stars	(0.0010)	(0.0006)	(4.7782)
Dummy = 1 if	1.3417‡	−0.3512‡	−225.45
entrant (firm	(0.1455)	(0.0733)	(163.82)
born >1975), else 0			
Years from entry	0.1209‡	0.0643‡	36.439
into biotech to 1989	(0.0191)	(0.0088)	(22.719)
(age)			
Dummy = 1 if firm	0.2845‡	−0.5880‡	267.78†
uses recombinant	(0.1278)	(0.0567)	(131.56)
DNA, else 0			
Inverse Mills ratio	n/a	n/a	166.33†
(selectivity			(74.189)
correction)			
Log-likelihood	−169.46	−296.20	n/a[b]
Log-likelihood coefs.	−255.28	−323.14	n/a[b]
= 0			

NOTE: All variables are for individual California firms responding to a telephone census on employment in 1994 ($N = 76$) except as noted. Standard errors are in parentheses below coefficients. Probability $|t\text{-stat}|>x$: *≤ 0.10, †≤ 0.05, ‡≤ 0.01.

a. Poisson regression for counts of the firm's products in development or on the market in 1990; standard errors are adjusted by Wooldridge's procedure 2.1 (Wooldridge 1991).

b. Second-stage Heckman estimates for nonzero 1989–1994 employment change observations with consistent variance-covariance matrix estimates (five); inverse Mills ratio is correction for selectivity (or response) bias for firms reporting no change from 1989; adjusted $R^2 = 0.1623$.

SOURCE: Adapted from Zucker, Darby, and Armstrong 1997a, tables 2 and 3.

FIGURE 7-2

PREDICTED PRODUCTS AND EMPLOYMENT GROWTH OF OTHERWISE
AVERAGE FIRM ACCORDING TO NUMBER OF ARTICLES WRITTEN BY
FIRM'S SCIENTISTS AND ACADEMIC STARS

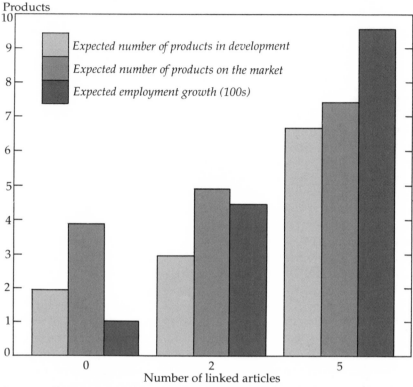

Expected number of products in development

Expected number of products on the market

Expected employment growth (100s)

Number of linked articles

SOURCE: Estimates in Zucker, Darby, and Armstrong, 1997a.

product in development, about one more product on the market, and
about 345 more employment growth from 1989 to 1994. For five such
articles, the effect was 4.7 more products in development, 3.5 more
products on the market, and about 860 more employees. Since these
employees are highly paid (averaging around $60,000 per year), the
effect on the local economy is substantial, with more than a $10 million
annual payroll increase per article.

Contrary to the predictions of advocates of geographically localized knowledge spillovers, articles written by academic stars positively
affect local firms only for those stars specifically linked to the firm, a
relationship indicating likely ownership, consulting arrangement, or
other market exchange. We believe that these scientist-entrepreneurs

55

use their valuable knowledge both to obtain resources for their research and to benefit financially from their discoveries. Because of the
extensive tacit knowledge involved in using and evaluating their discoveries, university intellectual-property managers indicate that few, if
any, technology transfer arrangements in biotechnology would occur
between the university and the firm unless one or more of the discovering scientists is personally involved in and gaining from the commercial application.

A real puzzle is why the numbers of articles by affiliated stars
have either an insignificant or a statistically significant but quite small
positive effect on our measures of a firm's success. We find similar
results in work underway for the United States and Japan and are
using those larger samples to explore the issue in more detail. We hy-
pothesize that an important role for these affiliated star scientists is
facilitating links with academic stars, and how well they do that is
picked up in the coefficients on the linked articles. Perhaps, too, affiliated stars are qualitatively different, but it is hard to argue that they
are not as good, since ever-affiliated stars on average have more than
twice the citations per year of ever-linked but never-affiliated stars
(who themselves have about a 50 percent higher citation rate than stars
with no detectable ties to firms). Possibly the stars who are willing to
leave the university for full-firm affiliation are more deeply involved in
production processes than product discovery.[12]

New entrants have significantly more products in development
and fewer on the market than incumbent firms. Employees of incumbent firms argue that they are better at killing losers and getting winners to market than the entrants are, who often have fewer research
alternatives. Given the nature of the product counts, however, this difference could simply reflect a strategy in which the entrants concentrate more on high-science products, which take longer for FDA
approval. That interpretation is consistent with the sign pattern for the
recombinant-DNA dummy variable, but that variable results in significantly higher predicted employment growth, while entrants have
insignificantly lower employment growth than incumbents. Age has
the expected positive effect on success.

As a whole, these results (and our research on the entire United

---

12. If affiliated stars work primarily in the production process rather than
in discovery, they would have little effect on products in development, would
speed up products on the market, and would have an ambiguous effect on
employment growth depending on whether any decrease in production cost
per unit increases output sufficiently to offset lower employment per unit associated with greater efficiency.

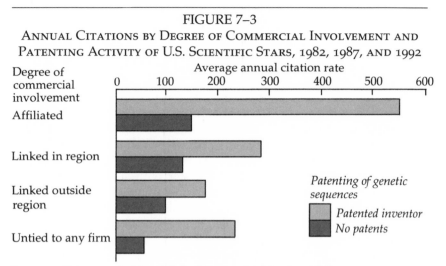

FIGURE 7–3

ANNUAL CITATIONS BY DEGREE OF COMMERCIAL INVOLVEMENT AND
PATENTING ACTIVITY OF U.S. SCIENTIFIC STARS, 1982, 1987, AND 1992

SOURCE: Data reported in table 1 of Zucker and Darby, 1996.

States and Japan) suggest that the strongest predictor of a successful biotech firm is the number of articles cowritten with an academic star scientist. Almost all the most successful biotech firms have such links and few firms that have them are not highly successful. One question is whether success leads to links (for trophy purposes) rather than the other way around, but Zucker, Darby, and Armstrong (1997a) report that these links are generally begun very early in the firm's history, in the case of already established scientists, or very early in the scientist's career for those who begin publishing after the firm's entry. Thus, either the firm or the scientist was not yet a success, and in either case the trophy hypothesis fails. Extensive interviews and other fieldwork lead us to believe that the linking impacts have real productivity effects and that they identify the firms that were started with active participation of outstanding academic scientists who combined genius and entrepreneurial spirit, often very early in the process of commercially applying the continuing scientific breakthroughs.

Commercial Involvement and the Scientific Productivity of Star Scientists

Zucker and Darby (1996) examine the effect of commercial involvement of stars on their scientific productivity. Figure 7–3 summarizes the data illustrating that the more scientists are involved in commercialization—whether in their publishing record, patenting activity, or both—the higher their average annual citations in the scientific literature. In fact, stars who have patented a gene sequence and are affiliated with a firm on at least one article have more than seven times the citation rate of the pure, academic star who has no patents and has never published a genetic sequence discovery up to 1990 as or with an employee of a U.S. firm.

The question is what causes the difference. In part, the difference seems to reflect the energy level (or entrepreneurialism) of the particular scientist: stars who have ever affiliated or are locally linked publish at a higher rate than do those who have never been linked to a firm or only to one outside the local region. The publication rate goes up again for stars who patent compared with a star with similar commercial involvement but no patents. We examined whether the publishing rate per year was higher before linking or affiliation with a firm on the hypothesis that increased secrecy might cut back publication. Instead, we found that the rate was actually higher, although the difference was not statistically significant, than before or after the period in which the publishing history indicates ties to a firm.

Possibly, any secrecy effects are offset by the greater resources available through ties to a firm, but it may also be that suppression of publication beyond the short period required for patenting is unlikely to be in the firm's interest: a major incumbent firm argues that a liberal publishing policy is important not to deter the best scientists from coming and to build the reputation necessary to attract other outstanding scientists, in addition to good citizenship in contributing to the common pool of science (Zucker and Darby 1997a). New entrants have all these motivations in addition to the need to prove themselves to venture capitalists and capital markets until their products finally reach the market to provide sufficient cash flow to keep the firm alive.

Higher citation rates per publication account for even more of the variation in total citations in figure 7–3 than do publication rates. Table 7–2 reports regressions that estimate whether the articles of stars who have ever been affiliated with or linked to a firm have higher rates of citation according to whether they were published before, during, or after the period of involvement with a firm (see also Zucker and Darby 1995). Articles by affiliated stars published during their affiliation have significantly higher rates of citation (about double) compared with their own record before and after affiliation and to that of stars untied to firms. This correlation holds for both world and U.S. data, while data for all stars show that stars linked to firms have significantly higher citation rates during that period of involvement with the firm. (If we use U.S. data, the estimated increase in citation rate is nearly as great, but it is not statistically significant in the smaller sample.) The only evidence of a selectivity effect (stars lucky enough to have a "hit"

TABLE 7–2
TOTAL CITATIONS TO ARTICLES BY STAR SCIENTISTS,
1982, 1987, AND 1992

Variables	Coefficients and standard errors	
	World	U.S. only
Constant	−31.676‡	−42.789‡
	(6.092)	(9.536)
STARAF = 1 if any star author lists a firm affiliation, else 0	17.671‡	20.915‡
	(4.024)	(7.076)
COLAF = 1 if any of collaborators lists a firm affiliation, else 0	7.626‡	5.254
	(2.428)	(3.585)
PREAF = 1 if for any star author year <1st-affiliated year, else 0	−1.983	3.661
	(2.257)	(4.362)
POSTAF = 1 if for any star author year ≥1st-affiliated year, else 0	−3.114	−6.644
	(2.844)	(5.943)
PRELK = 1 if for any star author year <1st-linked year, else 0	4.285‡	1.378
	(1.175)	(1.702)
POSTLK = 1 if for any star author year ≥1st-linked year, else 0	−3.114	−0.514
	(2.844)	(1.731)
Number of authors on the article	2.227‡	3.062‡
	(0.203)	(0.340)
Number of star authors on the article	2.519‡	0.942
	(0.679)	(1.095)
Year	4.994‡	6.707‡
	(0.727)	(1.112)
$(Year)^2$	−0.176‡	−0.229‡
	(0.022)	(0.033)
Adjusted R^2	0.106	0.133

NOTE: All variables refer to the authors and publication date of each of the articles written by one or more stars. Probability |t-stat|>x: * <.05, †<.01, ‡<.001.
SOURCE: Zucker and Darby 1995, table 5.

article getting the opportunity to be involved with firms) is found for stars linked to firms in the world sample.[13] Otherwise, the evidence points to increased citation rates for articles published during periods when stars are involved with firms compared either with their own prior and subsequent record or to that of stars untied to firms.

Taken together, the evidence indicates that very productive scientists are the ones most likely to become involved in commercializing

---

13. Contrary to the simpler hypothesis, however, their citation rate remains high during the period of involvement within the firm.

their discoveries, that their rate of publishing continues during involvement with the firm at that extraordinary rate, and that the scientific quality of the publications as judged by citations increases during involvement with the firm. Thus, contrary to our original and widely shared hypothesis, commercial involvement has proved to be a complement to rather than a substitute for scientific productivity and contribution to the common pool of scientific literature. Blumenthal, Causino, Campbell, and Louis (1996) and Rosenberg (1996) have expressed deep reservations that commercial support of medical research may result in increased secrecy and ultimately in lost lives. We cannot speak to clinical trials and comparative tests where the press has occasionally reported results suppressed for commercial reasons, but certainly our evidence suggests that in the discovery end of research, where our star scientists are likely to be involved, commercial involvement and patenting go hand in hand with very high if not increased rates of publication and with more important publications.

National Innovation Systems That Promote
Stars' Commercial Involvement

We have argued that in the case of biotechnology the U.S. national innovation system has performed very well: despite natural excludability based on extensive tacit knowledge, new technology has diffused rapidly; some of the best academic scientists have been entrepreneurially involved in commercialization of the scientific breakthroughs to the particular benefit of the communities in which their universities were located as well as the nation generally; and the stars who have gotten involved not only did well financially but also enhanced their scientific contributions, in some cases resulting in significant life-saving and life-enhancing new products. In the next stage of our research, we attempt to understand which aspects of our national innovation system worked well and which could be strengthened.

In Zucker and Darby (1997b), we begin to explore these issues by comparing the countries of the Asia-Pacific Economic Cooperation (APEC) forum and Europe.[14] Referring to figure 7–4, we note two unfavorable indicators for European conditions: (1) Europe (and the rest of the world) has negative net migration rates, losing stars to the APEC

14. We have found only four APEC countries in which star scientists have reported affiliations: the United States, Japan, Australia, and Canada. Stars have published in ten countries of the enlarged European Union plus Switzerland. The only rest-of-the-world countries with stars (up to 1990) were Israel and the USSR.

FIGURE 7–4
INTERNATIONAL COMPARISON OF THE IMPORTANCE OF UNIVERSITIES,
NET MIGRATION, AND COMMERCIAL INVOLVEMENT OF
STAR BIOSCIENTISTS

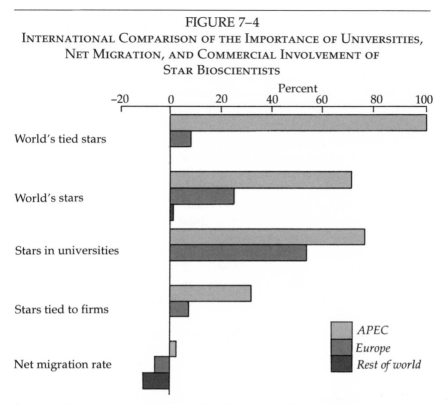

SOURCE: Data reported in tables 1–3 in Zucker and Darby 1997.

countries, particularly the United States and Japan; and (2) a much lower percentage of European stars (and no rest-of-the-world stars) is tied to firms (either affiliated with a firm or publishing with employees of a firm in their own country). That is, Europe has a much smaller share of the world's stars actively involved in commercialization than even its small (relative to population) share of the total stars. In sum, scientists are less likely to become stars in Europe, but if they do, they are more likely to leave and less likely to get their hands dirty working at the bench-level science with a firm's employees. While the gap in total numbers may be explained in part by greater funding and emphasis on basic research in the United States, the lack of high-level technology transfer makes a bad situation worse.

Thus, we must report that Europe offers those of us in America and Japan a cautionary tale and the challenge of figuring out what we were doing well before we make serious mistakes. One factor highlighted in figure 7–4 that we intend to investigate in future research is

61

the dominant role of research universities here and in Japan compared with much greater reliance on research institutes in other countries. The idea of research institutes sounds very attractive, particularly in a smaller country that sees them as a vehicle to achieve a critical mass by concentrating the nation's best scientists in one place. In fact, we ourselves would like to have our research well funded until retirement and the opportunity to build a more permanent research team without the need to train successive generations of graduate students and post-doctoral fellows. Despite the personal attractions, we can also see how that situation might cool the entrepreneurial spirit, particularly if one is seen as a truly full-time employee of the institute and therefore con-strained by various conflict-of-interest rules from profiting from any involvement or collaboration with firms.

Our future research will concentrate on international studies of the effects of alternative institutions, policies, and regulations on the creation and commercialization of the science base in biotechnology. These concerns are not merely historical but are rather motivated by the desire that we make the most of future breakthroughs, which create new or transform old science-driven high-technology industries.

Summary and Remaining Questions

The U.S. scientific infrastructure has performed well both in producing the revolution in bioscience and in commercializing the new technol-ogy. Years of patient investment through U.S. government funding, university resources, and the talents of individual researchers have paid off successfully. Bioscience was not an area particularly targeted for funding before the revolution started, but support was quickly stepped up afterward. As a result, the United States has benefited from having nearly two-thirds of the world's bioscience star scientists work here at some time and has approximately half the world's science base. Because biotechnology, like many other areas of science, involves much tacit knowledge, it is not easy for other countries to catch up simply by reading publications reporting these scientists' research.

Industrial applications developed mostly where the stars and major research universities were to begin with and, to a lesser extent, where the stars were attracted. The effects of the research break-throughs have an important geographically localized effect on eco-nomic growth and development. This local impact is due primarily to entrepreneurially inclined academic star scientists who see commer-cially important uses of their basic science discoveries and are person-ally involved in the firms' turning their vision into reality. The (usually part-time) personal participation of stars in working with the firm's scientists has resulted in widespread benefits: the firms with such involvement are much more successful, providing significant gains in highly paid employment for the communities around the stars' universities as well as more new products for the nation—products that in many cases have been life saving as well as life enhancing. Many star scientists have prospered, some becoming very wealthy, as a result of combining scientific genius with commercial entrepreneurship, but their scientific contributions have continued unabated in quantity while increasing in quality during the period of their commercial activity.

Although personal involvement of stars in commercializing their basic science discoveries played an important role in both scientific and commercial productivity, it was surprisingly rare outside the APEC countries (in particular, except for the United States and Japan). Our fieldwork and preliminary empirical analysis lead us to believe that institutions, laws, subsidies, and university policies have all played an important role in determining the degree of commercial ties between stars and firms.

Much more work is needed to sort out the quantitative importance of these factors. For example, how important to U.S. technology transfer is the generally permissive view of universities toward professors as principals in or consultants to firms? Are European-style subsidies to firms an effective substitute for merit-based research funding? What more can be said about how commercialization has affected the growth of bioscience? Are the results of this analysis generalizable to other technologies? Which ones? Only during the revolutionary phase after major scientific revolutions or at other times?

Successful research is identified more by the questions it raises than the answers it offers. One of the great pleasures of this research—besides being able to work with each other and our remarkable team of colleagues and students—is an exponentially growing list of questions that keeps delaying our ending the project and turning to something else.

Note

This research has been supported by grants from the Alfred P. Sloan Foundation through the NBER Research Program on Industrial Technology and Productivity, the National Science Foundation (SES 9012925), the University of California Systemwide Biotechnology Research and Education Program, and the University of California's Pacific Rim Research Program. This article builds on an ongoing project in which Marilynn B. Brewer also long played a leading role. Jeff Armstrong was responsible for the analysis of firm success and Maximo Torero for the APEC-Europe comparative analysis.

The authors are indebted to a remarkably talented team of post-doctoral fellows—Jeff Armstrong, Zhong Deng, Julia Liebeskind, and Yusheng Peng—and research assistants—Paul J. Alapat, Cherie Barba, Lynda J. Kim, Kerry Knight, Edmundo Murrugara, Amalya Oliver, Alan Paul, Richard Powell, Jane Ren, Erika Rick, Benedikt Stefansson, Yui Suzuki, Akio Tagawa, Maximo Torero, Melissa Van Dyck, Alan Wang, and Mavis Wu. This chapter is a part of the NBER's research program in productivity. Any opinions expressed are those of the authors and not those of the National Bureau of Economic Research.

References

Acs, Zoltan, David B. Audretsch, and Maryann P. Feldman. "Real Effects of Academic Research: Comment." *American Economic Review*, vol. 82, no. 1 (March 1992), pp. 363–67.

Arrow, Kenneth J. "Economic Welfare and the Allocation of Resources for Invention." In Richard R. Nelson, ed., *The Rate and Direction of Inventive Activity: Economic and Social Factors*, NBER Special Conference Series, vol. 13. Princeton, N.J.: Princeton University Press, 1962, pp. 609–25.

———. *The Limits of Organization*. New York, N.Y.: W.W. Norton & Company, 1974.

Blumenthal, David, Nancyanne Causino, Eric Campbell, and Karen Seashore Louis. "Relationships between Academic Institutions and Industry in the Life Sciences—An Industry Survey." *New England Journal of Medicine*, vol. 334, no. 6 (February 8, 1996), pp. 368–73.

Cohen, Stanley, A. Chang, Herbert Boyer, and R. Helling. "Construction of Biologically Functional Bacterial Plasmids *in vitro*." *Proceedings of the National Academy of Sciences*, vol. 70 (1973), pp. 3240–44.

Darby, Michael R., and Lynne G. Zucker. "Star Scientists, Institutions, and the Entry of Japanese Biotechnology Enterprises." National Bureau of Economic Research working paper no. 5795, October 1996.

Eisenberg, Rebecca S. "Proprietary Rights and the Norms of Science in Biotechnology Research." *Yale Law Journal*, vol. 97 (December 1987), pp. 177–231.

GenBank. Release 65.0, machine readable data base. Palo Alto, Calif.: IntelliGentics, Inc., September 1990.

————. Release 81.0, machine readable data base. Bethesda, Md.: National Center for Biotechnology Information, February 15, 1994.

Griliches, Zvi. "Hybrid Corn: An Exploration in the Economics of Technological Change." *Econometrica*, vol. 25, no. 4 (October 1957), pp. 501–22.

Jaffe, Adam B. "Real Effects of Academic Research." *American Economic Review*, vol. 79, no. 5 (December 1989), pp. 957–70.

Jaffe, Adam B., Manuel Trajtenberg, and Rebecca Henderson. "Geographic Localization of Knowledge Spillovers as Evidenced by Patent Citations." *Quarterly Journal of Economics*, vol. 63, no. 3 (August 1993), pp. 577–98.

Liebeskind, Julia Porter, Amalya Lumerman Oliver, Lynne G. Zucker, and Marilynn B. Brewer. "Social Networks, Learning, and Flexibility: Sourcing Scientific Knowledge in New Biotechnology Firms." *Organization Science*, vol. 7, no. 4 (July/August 1996), pp. 428–43.

Nelson, Richard R. "The Simple Economics of Basic Scientific Research." *Journal of Political Economy*, vol. 67, no. 3 (June 1959), pp. 297–306.

Nelson, Richard R., and Sidney G. Winter. *An Evolutionary Theory of Economic Change.* Cambridge, Mass.: Harvard University Press, 1982.

Rosenberg, Nathan. *Inside the Black Box: Technology and Economics.* Cambridge: Cambridge University Press, 1982.

Rosenberg, Steven A. "Sounding Board: Secrecy in Medical Research." *New England Journal of Medicine*, vol. 334, no. 6 (February 8, 1996), pp. 392–94.

Sindelar, Robert D. "Overview/Preview of Current and Future Recombinant DNA-Produced Pharmaceuticals." *Drug Topics*, April 20, 1992, supplement, pp. 3–16.

————. "The Pharmacy of the Future." *Drug Topics*, vol. 137, no. 9 (May 21, 1993), pp. 66–84.

Wooldridge, Jeffrey M. "On the Application of Robust, Regression-based Diagnostics to Models of Conditional Means and Conditional Variances." *Journal of Econometrics*, vol. 47 (January 1991), pp. 5–46.

Zucker, Lynne G., Marilynn B. Brewer, Amalya Oliver, and Julia Liebeskind. "Basic Science as Intellectual Capital in Firms: Information Dilemmas in rDNA Biotechnology Research." Working paper, UCLA Institute for Social Science Research, 1993.

Zucker, Lynne G., and Michael R. Darby. "Virtuous Circles of Productivity: Star Bioscientists and the Institutional Transformation of Industry." National Bureau of Economic Research working paper no. 5342, November 1995.

65

———. "Star Scientists and Institutional Transformation: Patterns of Invention and Innovation in the Formation of the Biotechnology Industry." *Proceedings of the National Academy of Sciences*, vol. 93, no. 23 (November 12, 1996), pp. 12709–716.

———. "Present at the Revolution: Transformation of Technical Identity for a Large Incumbent Pharmaceutical Firm after the Biotechnological Breakthrough." *Research Policy*, 1997a, forthcoming.

———. "Star Scientist Linkages to Firms in APEC and European Countries: Indicators of Regional Institutional Differences Affecting Competitive Advantage." *International Journal of Technology Management*, 1997b, forthcoming.

Zucker, Lynne G., Michael R. Darby, and Jeff Armstrong. "Intellectual Capital and the Firm: The Technology of Geographically Localized Knowledge Spillovers." National Bureau of Economic Research working paper no. 4946, December 1994.

———. "Intellectual Human Capital and the Firm: The Technology of Geographically Localized Knowledge Spillovers." *Economic Inquiry*, 1997a, forthcoming.

———. "Sources of Superior Performing Firms: Evidence from the U.S. Biotechnology Industry." Working paper, UCLA Institute for Social Science Research, February 1997b.

Zucker, Lynne G., Michael R. Darby, and Marilynn B. Brewer. "Intellectual Capital and the Birth of U.S. Biotechnology Enterprises." National Bureau of Economic Research working paper no. 4653, February 1994.

———. "Intellectual Human Capital and the Birth of U.S. Biotechnology Enterprises." *American Economic Review*, vol. 87, no. 4 (September 1997), forthcoming.

Zucker, Lynne G., Michael R. Darby, Marilynn B. Brewer, and Yusheng Peng. "Collaboration Structure and Information Dilemmas in Biotechnology: Organizational Boundaries as Trust Production." In Roderick M. Kramer and Tom R. Tyler, eds., *Trust in Organizations*. Thousand Oaks, Calif.: Sage, 1996, pp. 90–113.

8

Commentary: Shoring Up Government Support

Frank R. Lichtenberg

Varmus, Kornberg, and Zucker and Darby raise a number of interesting and important questions about government support of biomedical research. The total amount of government-funded health research has increased substantially in real terms over the past thirty years, but noncommercial health research as a percentage of total health expenditure was more than twice as high in 1965 as it has been in the 1990s (see figure 8–1). During the same period, private research expenditure as a percentage of sales of R&D–performing manufacturing companies *increased* by more than 50 percent (see figure 8–2). The decline in noncommercial health R&D intensity is not necessarily a cause for concern, for several reasons. First, this decline may be attributable to "excessive" growth in the denominator of this ratio, national health expenditure. The diffusion of managed care may have begun to curb this possibly "excessive" growth in the mid- to late 1980s. (The decline in noncommercial health R&D intensity essentially halted in 1985.)[1] Second, during the past thirty years, *industry*-sponsored health R&D has increased much more rapidly than national health expenditure: the ratio of the former to the latter increased from 1.1 percent in 1965 to 1.8 percent in 1993. But the increase in private health–R&D intensity has offset less than half the reduction in government health–R&D in-

---

1. However, as Glenn Hubbard argues in his article, the substitution of managed care for traditional fee-for-service medicine has probably resulted in increased financial distress of academic medical centers, possibly reducing their ability to engage in biomedical R&D.

FIGURE 8–1

NONCOMMERCIAL HEALTH RESEARCH AS A PERCENTAGE OF
NATIONAL HEALTH EXPENDITURE, 1965–1994

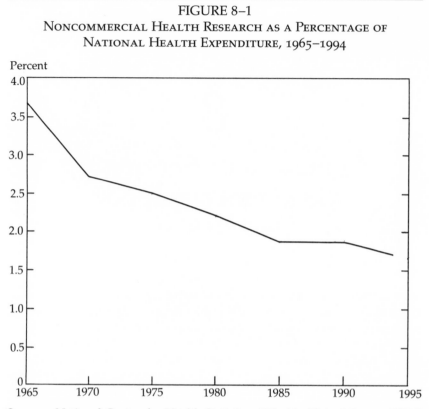

SOURCE: National Center for Health Statistics, "Health, United States, 1995."
Hyattsville, Md.: 1996, table 119.

tensity, so that total health R&D intensity declined from 4.6 percent in
1965 to 3.5 percent in 1993. Moreover, private research is likely to be
more targeted, and less "basic," than government research. Kornberg
argues that, because major medical discoveries are commonly serendipitous, "success requires channeling a major fraction of the budget
into noncategorical, basic research."

Varmus highlights the problem of instability of government-
funded biomedical R&D. As figure 8–3 indicates, his concern appears
to be well founded: the growth in federal health R&D expenditure has
been quite volatile over the past two decades. Periods of rapid growth
are followed by periods of low nominal growth (probably periods of
negative real growth). Spending, for example, increased by 11.6 percent from 1984 to 1985, by 1.5 percent the following year, and by 13.8
percent from 1986 to 1987. Instability of biomedical R&D funding

68

FIGURE 8–2
COMPANY-FUNDED R&D SPENDING AS A PERCENTAGE OF SALES,
1957–1993

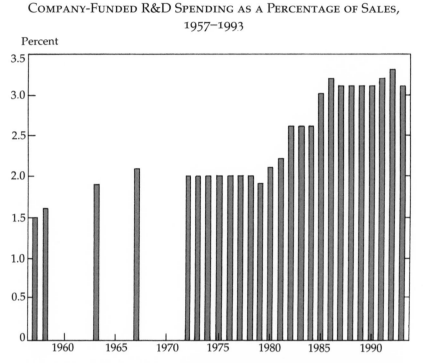

SOURCE: National Science Foundation, "Research and Development in Industry: 1993." NSF 96-304. Washington, D.C.: NSF, 1994 and previous years.

is likely to reduce the productivity of (or social returns to) this expenditure.

The federal government's ability to sponsor biomedical research
might be enhanced if it appropriated a larger fraction of the social returns to its innovations. Varmus reports that NIH earns only about $20
million per year from royalties for inventions. This is about 0.2 percent
of its annual research expenditures. In contrast, my employer, Columbia University, whose total research budget is much smaller than
NIH's, received $40.7 million in license revenue from 253 active license
agreements in 1995–1996.[2] Kornberg has definite and provocative ideas
about how government biomedical research resource allocation decisions should (and should not) be made. He argues that these decisions
should be made mainly or even exclusively on the basis of scientific

2. In terms of licensing revenues received, Columbia is one of the top three
universities in the United States (Columbia University 1997).

FIGURE 8–3
ANNUAL PERCENTAGE CHANGE IN FEDERAL HEALTH R&D
EXPENDITURE, 1975–1993

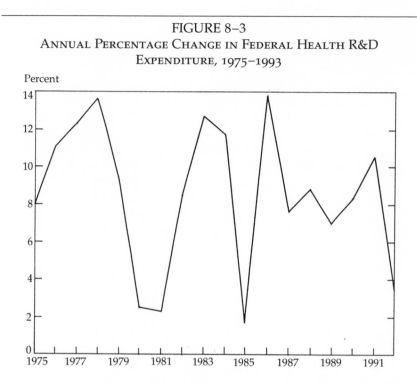

SOURCE: National Center for Health Statistics, "Health, United States, 1995."
Hyattsville, Md.: Public Health Service, 1996, table 131.

curiosity: certain research projects should receive government support merely because scientists are curious about the ideas, even if there is no prospect of economic or social benefit from the research. Kornberg favors this policy not because he is indifferent to the economic or social benefits of research, but because he believes that the ultimate benefits of a given project are almost completely unpredictable. This unpredict-ability is due, in part, to the typically considerable lag between inven-tion and commercial exploitation: "Time and again, inventors created things that had to wait many years to be recognized for their practical value." He cites numerous examples to support his claim that "investi-gations that seemed totally irrelevant to any practical objective have yielded most of the major discoveries of medicine." Indeed, "the pur-suit of curiosity about the basic facts of nature has proven throughout the history of medical science to be the most practical, the most *cost-effective* route to successful drugs and devices."[3] This view is echoed

---

3. In a recent econometric study, Andrew Toole estimated that a 10 percent

by Ralph Gomory, president of the Alfred P. Sloan Foundation, who likes to say that it is possible to guarantee that a scientific discovery is useful, but it is impossible to guarantee that a discovery is *not* (or will never be) useful.

Kornberg argues that society will ultimately realize greater benefits from biomedical research spending if government officials refrain from attempting to achieve specific objectives—micro- or even macro-managing the research budget—such as finding a cure for cancer or AIDS. He is hostile to the notion of a strategic plan for biomedical research, which was advocated by the former director of NIH: "The best plan over many decades has been no plan."[4]

This view suggests that there may be serious political difficulties associated with public support of biomedical research. The public and their elected representatives expect recipients of government funds to be *accountable* for how those funds are used. Kornberg argues that, to a significant degree, scientists cannot and should not be held accountable for the government funds that they receive to conduct their research. Provided that they demonstrate a reasonable level of curiosity (and presumably also competence), scientists need merely to say "trust me" to the government for the latter to honor their funding requests.

Kornberg is certainly correct that public biomedical R&D resource allocation decisions should not be made *entirely* on the basis of the relative burden of various diseases. And Congress frequently attempts to pressure the NIH to concentrate its research efforts on a particular disease (which critics refer to as the disease of the month). But R&D allocation decisions should not be completely independent of, or unrelated to, relative disease burden either. In a recent paper, I have developed a simple model of optimal R&D resource allocation that indicates that the socially optimal amount of R&D expenditure related to a particular disease should depend positively on both the relative burden of the disease and the relative degree of scientific opportunity, or research productivity, in that area of research (Lichtenberg 1997). In other words, the efficient level of R&D spending depends on both the demand for and the supply (or cost) of innovations. Consequently,

---

increase in Public Health Service basic research funding leads, on average, to a 22–25 percent increase in the number of FDA-approved new chemical entities (NCEs), but with a lag of approximately twenty years. A 10 percent increase in pharmaceutical industry R&D funding leads to only about a 7 percent increase in NCEs approved, with a much shorter lag.

4. Some have an analogous view about parenting. Children of parents who attempt to guide and control their children's development closely may turn out to be less successful than children whose parents are more *laissez-faire*.

even though a certain disease may impose a large burden on society, it may not be worthy of high relative research funding if the relative productivity of expenditure on research on that disease is low. The relative *demand* for a cure of, or relief from, a disease is relatively easy to measure: government statistics reveal how many people suffer from a disease, are limited in activity or die from it, etc.[5] In contrast, relative scientific opportunity is extremely difficult to measure, at least by non-scientists (including politicians). This is why, I think, Kornberg believes that research allocation decisions should be left entirely up to scientists. In a sense, Zucker and Darby subscribe to an even more extreme view of the degree of privacy (or cost of transmitting) scientific information. They argue that scientific knowledge is so tacit that even scientists outside of the lab in which a discovery is made (let alone politicians) will fail to comprehend it fully even if it is described in publications.

There appears to be a fundamental disagreement between Kornberg and Zucker-Darby about the relationship between the pursuit of basic scientific knowledge and the commercial or practical application and exploitation of that knowledge. Kornberg is concerned about the prospect of scientists (particularly young ones) being seduced by commercial ventures, since the latter tend to pursue "safe and practical projects over the untried and adventurous" (because "the process of invention conflicts with prudent business strategy"). But Zucker and Darby conclude from their detailed and extensive study of the biotechnology field that commercial involvement is a complement rather than a substitute for scientific productivity: commercial involvement and patenting go hand in hand with high rates of publication and citation. They find that the scientific productivity of stars is higher during their period of involvement with firms and that there is substantial congruence among stars' scientific goals, their financial goals, and firms' commercial goals.

References

Columbia University. 1997. *Columbia Innovation Enterprise Annual Report—Fiscal Year 1995/96.* New York: Columbia.

Lichtenberg, Frank. 1997. "The Allocation of Publicly Funded Biomedical Research." Unpublished papers. Columbia University.

---

5. Preliminary estimates suggest that the amount of public research about a disease is positively related to the number of deaths from that disease and the number of people who are limited in activity by it but is unrelated to simple prevalence of that disease (the number of people who report that they suffer from the disease).

PART THREE
Long-Term Funding Challenges for Biomedical Research

9

Federal Funding of R&D in an Era of Budgetary Restraint

June E. O'Neill and Philip C. Webre

No one can know what the future holds for federal outlays on research and development. As part of the discretionary budget, research and development (R&D) has no permanent spending authority and is, instead, subject to annual appropriations. If recent history is a guide, however, a squeeze on total discretionary spending is likely to be an important element of any short-term or long-term effort to balance the budget. Because the future of R&D spending is linked to budget developments, we will comment briefly on those developments before elaborating on the R&D budget.

At present, the federal budget deficit appears to be relatively tame, having declined to $107 billion in fiscal year 1996, or only about 1.4 percent of the gross domestic product (figure 9–1). Moreover the Congressional Budget Office (CBO) expects the deficit, after declining still further in 1997, to rise only modestly over the next decade under current laws and policies. But the outlook deteriorates dramatically after 2010, when the huge baby-boom generation will begin to retire and draw benefits from the government's three biggest entitlement programs: Social Security, Medicare, and Medicaid. At the same time, growth in revenues will slow because the proportion of people working and paying taxes will shrink. As a result, the deficit will start to mount rapidly after 2010.[1]

If no actions are taken to change policy, the annual deficit and

---

1. For estimates of the long-term budget problem and options for dealing with it, see Congressional Budget Office, *Long-term Budgetary Pressures and Policy Options* (Washington, D.C.: Government Printing Office, March 1997).

FIGURE 9–1
THE DEFICIT AS A PERCENTAGE OF GDP, FISCAL YEARS 1930–2007

Percent

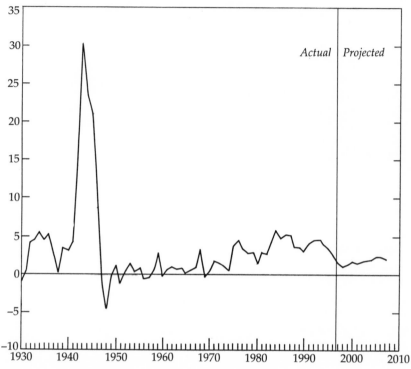

NOTE: Negative numbers indicate a budget surplus.
SOURCE: Congressional Budget Office and *Budget of the United States Government: Historical Tables.*

total debt will grow faster than GDP, setting in motion a vicious cycle with damaging feedback to the economy. Under those circumstances, current budget policy is unsustainable: in about four decades, the federal debt will exceed levels that the economy can support. Thus, at some point, the growth in federal outlays will have to be reduced, or taxes raised, or both. Because the costs of the required budgetary measures rise steeply with years of delay, there is strong reason to begin addressing our long-term budgetary problems now.

Balancing the Budget and Prospects for R&D

In May 1997, Congress and President Clinton reached a bipartisan agreement on a plan to balance federal outlays and revenues by the year 2002. Congress subsequently passed a budget resolution consistent with that agreement. Both the agreement and the budget resolution would slow the rate of growth of outlays enough to allow revenues—net of a tax cut—to catch up to outlays, yielding a small budget surplus in 2002.

Although growth in total federal outlays would slow under the budget agreement, after adjusting for inflation they are still projected to be slightly larger in 2002 than they are today. The discretionary component of spending, however, has not been spared. Total outlays for those programs will rise by less than the rate of inflation in each year of the agreement. In nominal terms, outlays for all discretionary programs would be only marginally larger in 2002 than in 1998, resulting in a real decline of 11 percent.

Budget negotiators have also agreed on measures to reduce the growth of outlays on entitlement programs, particularly Medicare and Medicaid. Nonetheless, entitlement spending will continue to outpace inflation by a large margin even after implementing the budget savings agreed on. Measured in dollars, however, the savings from curtailing the growth of entitlement spending are approximately equal to those obtained from imposing a near freeze in discretionary programs.

R&D Funding in the Past Two Decades. How will the future path of discretionary spending affect federal support for research and development? Over the past twenty years, federal R&D spending (excluding facilities) has slightly increased its share of discretionary outlays—from 11 percent in 1976 to an estimated 13 percent in 1996. Over that time period, total discretionary spending tripled in nominal dollar terms although declining as a share of federal outlays—and even rose by 20 percent after adjusting for inflation. In other words, R&D maintained a slightly increasing share of an increasing pie.

Although the discretionary pie has grown over the past twenty years, that growth has not been uniform over the whole period (figure 9–2). In fact, since 1991, when the Budget Enforcement Act first imposed caps on discretionary spending, such outlays fell by more than 12 percent after adjusting for inflation. During this more recent period, real (inflation-adjusted) R&D outlays have been on a roller coaster—rising and falling and rising and falling, before ending up slightly below the level where they started (figure 9–3). During the past decade and a half, defense and nondefense R&D expenditures moved in opposite directions. After doubling between 1978 and 1989, real defense R&D did not even keep up with inflation in the 1990s. By contrast, nondefense R&D, which had been roughly equal to defense R&D, fell by 30 percent in the early 1980s but has generally outpaced inflation since then. Those trends mirror the trends in total defense and nondefense discretionary spending.

77

FIGURE 9–2
DISCRETIONARY SPENDING, 1962–1996

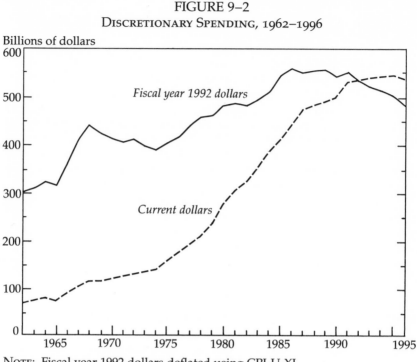

Billions of dollars

NOTE: Fiscal year 1992 dollars deflated using CPI-U-XI.
SOURCE: Congressional Budget Office.

If future budgets follow the paths laid out in the recent agreement for balancing the budget over the next five years, total discretionary spending will rise by 2 percent in nominal terms through 2002, implying a decline of 11 percent in real terms. Under those circumstances, the discretionary budget will be close to a zero-sum game. If future administrations and Congresses wish to expand certain programs significantly, they will have to reduce others. New initiatives could crowd out old programs. If the National Institutes of Health is to continue its recent nominal growth of 6 percent to 7 percent a year, for example, other agencies—possibly including other science agencies—will have to shrink.

Although nondefense R&D has fared relatively well during the virtual freeze on discretionary spending since 1991, the outlook is likely to be gloomier. Defense spending bore the brunt of the freeze, falling 17 percent in nominal terms, while domestic discretionary outlays actually rose by more than 25 percent. The ending of the cold war, however, facilitated the decline in defense spending, and that decline

FIGURE 9–3
FEDERAL RESEARCH AND DEVELOPMENT SPENDING, 1962–1998

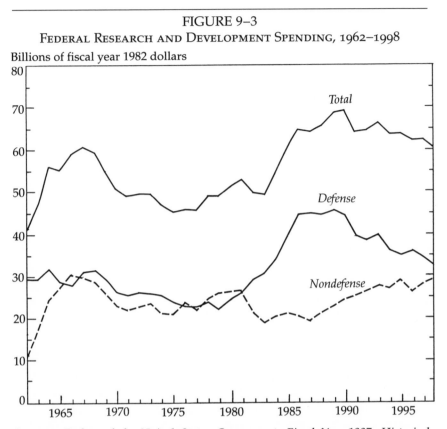

Billions of fiscal year 1982 dollars

SOURCE: *Budget of the United States Government, Fiscal Year 1997: Historical Tables.*

is coming to an end. In the congressional budget resolution for fiscal year 1998, both defense spending and nondefense spending are held to a 2 percent rise in nominal terms between 1997 and 2002.

R&D Funding in 1997 Appropriations and the 1998 Budget Resolution. The appropriations bills for fiscal year 1997 that the Congress passed last year reflect in nascent form many of the policy tensions and trade-offs among the various categories of discretionary spending, including R&D. Those appropriation bills boost total federal spending for R&D in 1997 to $74 billion in nominal terms, an increase from the 1996 level of 3.5 percent, which is somewhat more than the expected inflation rate (table 9–1). The 1997 rise in total federal spending for R&D, however, is spread unevenly among major categories. Defense R&D increases by 4.7 percent, but nondefense R&D by just 2.1 percent.

79

TABLE 9–1
1997 R&D Appropriations and the 1998 Request
(budget authority, in billions)

	1996 Actual	1997 Estimated	1998 President's Request
R&D Total	71.3	73.8	75.5
Defense	38.5	40.3	40.5
Nondefense	32.9	33.6	35.0

Note: Includes facilities and equipment.
Source: Office of Management and Budget.

Within the nondefense category, health research, which accounts for 40 percent of total nondefense R&D, grows at an annual rate of 7.4 percent. That leaves the burden of adjustment to fall more heavily on the R&D budgets of civilian agencies not involved in health.

The congressional commitment to health R&D also drives this year's 2.7 percent increase in funding for basic research. According to tallies by the American Association for the Advancement of Science, increases in basic research funding at the National Institutes of Health account for more than 100 percent of all increases received by basic research programs. Funding for basic research in non–health-related areas is down by 0.3 percent.

One consequence of the 1997 increase in defense R&D is a shift away from basic and applied research and toward product development. Should the new priority given to defense continue, those trends will also be likely to continue.

The recently passed budget resolution gives some early indication of Congress's intent with regard to R&D in the budget agreement. Within the budget functions that encompass most nondefense R&D—space and general science, energy, and health—discretionary outlays are up by 1.5 percent for 1998. But then they are scheduled to decrease by 4.5 percent by 2002 in nominal terms. How these cuts will be accommodated among R&D and non-R&D programs is not clear. In some instances, the R&D programs are such a large fraction of the function total that a cut in the function will necessarily mean a cut in the R&D program, unless there are extremely deep cuts in the non-R&D programs. In the defense area, total outlays are down slightly. Whether this will be translated into cuts in defense R&D is not yet known.

Implications for the Future

In assessing the broader impact of these changes in the federal budget for R&D, we should keep in mind that spending cuts are generally

FIGURE 9–4

RESEARCH AND DEVELOPMENT SPENDING, 1952–1996

Billions of 1987 dollars

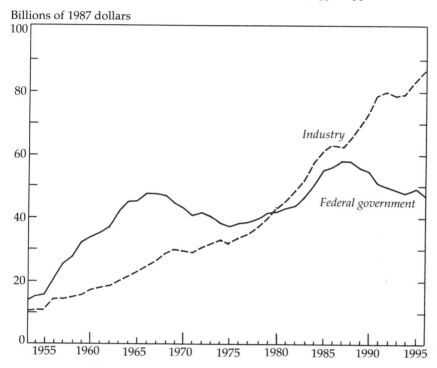

NOTE: Industrial R&D includes all nonfederal sources of industrial research and development funding.
SOURCE: National Science Foundation.

being made in the expectation that reducing the deficit will benefit the U.S. economy by increasing saving and investment. CBO's projections show that reductions in the budget deficit will make resources available to other actors in the economy, who, in turn, can be expected to boost *their* investment in R&D.

Indeed, for thirty-five years, private industry has been increasing its funding of R&D—both in real dollar terms and relative to federal agencies—despite a recent temporary pause. Since 1960, industry has almost quintupled its spending on R&D, even after inflation is taken into account (figure 9–4). In 1960, the federal government spent almost twice as much as industry on R&D, but, by 1996, it was spending just 55 percent of the private-sector level. There was a pause in the growth of private R&D in the early 1990s, perhaps even a slight decline in real terms after 1992. But that pause was probably related to the recession;

in fact, preliminary data from the National Science Foundation suggest that private R&D increased substantially over the past two years.

Federal cutbacks, especially if accompanied by renewed private R&D spending, will accelerate the trend of increasing reliance on the private sector to make the nation's investments in research and development. A greater shift to private-sector funding of R&D is likely to put more emphasis on applied research and product development and less on basic research.

Implications for Policy

With reliance on the private sector increasing, it will be more critical than ever for federal policy makers to seek the maximum social benefit from federal research dollars. The first step in doing so is to ensure that the federal effort underlying the R&D is appropriate—meaning that the research and development is expected to yield significant public benefits and would not otherwise be funded, or funded adequately, by private sources.

In some instances—such as defense and space R&D—the federal government is the primary user of the research and, therefore, is in a position to have both the knowledge of its needs and the incentive to see that they are met. In other cases, the line between appropriate and inappropriate areas for federal funding is less clear. Health research, for example, has generally produced large public benefits. Yet, high private returns in some areas, such as pharmaceutical research, have induced the private sector to undertake much of the research. But other aspects of health research—particularly more risky basic research—might not be undertaken without federal funding. With the proper incentives, such as appropriate intellectual property rights (including patent, trademark, and copyright laws) or a flexible regulatory structure, the private sector can be encouraged to play a greater role in providing R&D.

Unfortunately, although economics provides broad guidance, it can offer little concrete information to help the government make difficult choices about R&D. The simple maxim of economics—to invest in those projects with the highest marginal rate of return to society—may not be of much practical value to policy makers choosing among basic research projects, where the marginal rate of return is unknown and probably unknowable. Moreover, the academic fields and projects most likely to produce the kinds of short-term benefits that economists have been able to measure are precisely those that can most easily find support from private industry or venture capital markets.

Other academic fields—such as astronomy—have not produced

the types of short-term economic benefits that attract funding by industry, but they either balance out our intellectual portfolio or, as a former director of Fermilab is reputed to have observed, they "make the country worth defending." Which is to say, although the government's investment in those fields is comparatively small, it must be justified on the basis of intrinsic interest to society rather than as a direct economic contribution. Such research often plays a vital role in training students, who may then go on to make practical contributions of their own. And such research may eventually turn out to have a payoff. Given the history of the past hundred years, which of us can say with certainty that a given piece of knowledge will never be of practical use.

The choices to be made about which research projects to fund will become more difficult as time goes on and as the funds available for discretionary R&D grow scarcer. Congress and other science policy makers will continue to grapple with the question of how best to deploy this country's scarce R&D resources for the greatest benefit to society.

10

Emerging Issues and the Impact of Balancing the Federal Budget

Albert A. Barber

In collecting my thoughts on this subject, I looked through some of my material on funding requirements and emerging research issues that I accumulated during nearly forty years of research and research administration at UCLA. During the 1950s and 1960s, there did not seem to be many burning issues. We did the research, and the policy makers came up with the resources. I suppose that is why we now look on that time as the golden years of federally sponsored research.

In the 1970s, however, three emerging issues attracted our attention. The first was declining resources. We stayed fairly flat budgeted for the entire decade. The second was the explosive growth of audits. Federal auditors crawled all over our financial systems. The third was indirect cost as we moved from the earlier formula-based system to the cost-recovery system we presently use. The impact of these issues on the university was captured in the 1977 book by Smith and Karlesky, *The State of Academic Science*. It was also captured in the several reports published by the National Commission on Research. These issues of the 1970s that engaged us, therefore, were declining resources, the indirect cost of research, and the proliferation of federal audits.

In the 1980s, there were two sets of emerging issues. One set related to the increased interest in collaboration with industry, especially between our molecular biologists and their colleagues in biotechnology. Within this set were the issues of intellectual property, use of university facilities, conflicts of interest, research openness, and student independence. The second set related to the proliferation of federal regulations into the various social and ethical issues raised by academic research and researchers. Within this group were the issues of the use of animal subjects, the use of human subjects, the use of recombinant DNA, the use of hazardous materials, and scientific integrity. We were certainly never at a loss at identifying emerging issues during the 1980s.

In the 1990s, we still have all the issues that developed in the 1970s and the 1980s. We never get rid of issues. We simply look at them as continuing issues with new twists rather than as emerging issues. Regarding long-term funding for biomedical research, for example, we have addressed the continuing issue of resource constraints but within the context of the crises, opportunities, and economics of 1997 instead of those of the 1970s and 1980s. Resources will always be an issue since the crises, opportunities, and economics on which the support for research depends are always changing. We are looking at intellectual property and open scientific communication, issues that will continue as long as university-industry collaboration exists and is expanding to new universities, new disciplines, and new industries. New issues continue to emerge, such as genetic therapies and mammalian cloning.

Out of this smorgasbord of emerging and continuing research policy issues, I will focus on the issue of balancing the long-term need for federal science and technology resources as the president and Congress seek to balance the federal budget in the next five years. My comments will both complement and extend the chapter by O'Neill and Webre. When the discussions of balanced budgets started some three years ago, we were talking about a $300,000 billion per year annual deficit and predicting up to a 30–35 percent decrease, including losses to inflation, of the federal R&D budgets over a seven-year period. The deficit and the predicted cuts look considerably different now, but I did look at the potential impact of the earlier predicted cuts on the research programs of the University of California. I looked at both across-the-board cuts and selective agency cuts.

For the University of California, each 1 percent across-the-board cut is a loss of $13 million and, assuming an average of $200,000 per award, each 1 percent cut is a loss of some 65 awards. A 10 percent cut is a loss of $130 million and 650 awards. Given the political environment of 1994, selective cuts looked more realistic than did the across-the-board cuts, so I looked at UC awards by agencies. The Department of Energy cuts being discussed at that time devastated UC programs in fields as diverse as nuclear medicine, high-energy physics, radiobiology, fusion research, and environmental sciences. The Department of Commerce cuts severely affected the oceanography and climatology research programs at Scripps. National Aeronautics and Space Administration cuts affected the space sciences programs at the Los Angeles, Berkeley, and San Diego campuses. The Department of Defense cuts did their damage primarily to our engineering and computer science programs. One interesting number that fell out of this exercise was that if federal research support to UC was immediately cut by 35 percent and if we kept the same budgets for NIH and NSF, all research support from the other eleven federal agencies that support UC research disappears.

With two years of experience behind us, we can move away from predictions and look at some real numbers. The federal contract and grant awards to UC decreased about 4 percent between FY 1995 and FY 1996, and this trend seems to be continuing in the first quarter of FY 1997. National Institutes of Health awards, conversely, increased modestly from $670 million to $696 million, an increase of about 4 percent. The sum of awards from all non-NIH federal agencies decreased from $644 million to $560 million, a drop of 13 percent. NIH awards, therefore, were 59 percent of all federal awards to UC in FY 1996, up from 55 percent in FY 1995. In FY 1996, DOE was down 20 percent, Commerce was down 27 percent, DOD was down 7 percent, and NASA stayed the same. The important point is that even though the bottom line did not shift dramatically, the cuts did have a major impact on selected campus programs. These numbers are consistent with those reported in January by the National Academy of Sciences panel on federal science and technology (FS&T) analysis. That panel reported losses in constant dollars in the S&T budgets of all federal agencies except NIH and the National Science Foundation between FY 1994 and FY 1997. This report led to the recent statement by twenty-three scientific organizations recommending a 7 percent increase in all federal S&T budgets for FY 1998. Their position is not that NIH is overfunded but that the cuts being taken by other agencies are detrimental to our long-range FS&T needs. We all agree that biomedical research needs a long-term solution to funding needs. I hope that we would also agree that all federal science and technology research needs a long-term solution to the funding needs.

The FY 1996 agency budget actions were reflected in the awards to specific disciplines in the University of California. I suppose one would expect this, given the size of UC. The health and biological sciences receive increases that reflected the FY 1996 NIH increases. The physical sciences, however, were down nearly 20 percent and reflected the losses incurred by DOD, DOE, and, to some extent, NSF. Again, the UC experience is consistent with the disciplinary findings of the National Academy panel on the FS&T budget. My recommendation is that the entire FS&T budget be increased and be brought into balance so that we can meet the full range of educational and social challenges facing this nation. As we address this issue and as others attempt to balance the federal budget by the year 2002, I offer two modest proposals.

My first proposal is that we develop a specific educational program that effectively makes the case for the increases that we seek in the FS&T budget. The recent request from the scientific community for a 7 percent increase is an important step but probably not sufficient. As scientists, we have an outstanding story to tell, but we do not tell it well. We do it moderately well in connecting health research with treating disease and promoting well-being. We do it moderately well when we connect agriculture research to the food and fiber needs of the country. We do not do it well, however, in connecting geophysical research with earthquake prediction or in connecting meteorological research with climate prediction. We do not do it well in connecting materials research with advances in computing and communications. The list of examples where we do not do well is endless. We must mount a sustained effort to develop and communicate appropriate materials that demonstrate the connections between the research that is supported by the full range of FS&T budgets and the public benefits that accrue from that research. Developing good material is but half the loaf. The effective communication of the material to our public patrons and their elected representatives is the other, and probably the more important half. This is an urgent task, and we need to get at it if we are to have our voices heard as the policy makers grapple with ways to balance the federal budget.

My second proposal deals with the issue of strategic research. We must begin explaining that academic research is not simply some sort of a curiosity-driven activity but is of strategic importance to the entire federal science and technology agenda. We must convince the media to stop describing academic research in sound bites that come out something like "the federal government giving money to university researchers to pursue their own curiosity." Budget cuts tend to lead agencies to focus on short-term goals. Some, like NASA and DOD, will be forced to place a higher percentage of their resources into hardware commitments that already exist. It is, therefore, essential that the strategic importance of academic research for achieving the long-range federal S&T goals be clearly communicated. Also, the strategic importance of academic research must be effectively communicated to the federal agencies as they begin responding to the Government Performance and Results Act of 1993. In response to the act, agencies have been asked to set outcome-oriented goals and to measure progress in

87

achieving those goals. Under the banner of reinventing government, this appears to be another call for agencies to increase their portfolio of "strategic" research. I fear that an activity that is described as "university researchers pursuing their own curiosity" simply does not sell as an outcome-oriented goal.

Three points demonstrate the strategic nature of academic research, and once again I turn to UC data. The first, and most obvious one, is that 85 percent of the support for research at UC comes from federal agencies with clearly defined missions. The strategic importance of academic research is contained in the thousands of proposals and reports submitted by academic researchers to these agencies. The second point is that academic research is strategically important for investigating the full array of complex societal problems being addressed by federal agencies. These include problems related to energy production and conservation, communications, environmental changes, poverty, family stability, drug abuse, and global economic competitiveness. The list goes on. These researchers are not pursuing their own curiosity; they are applying their highly developed curiosity and talent in important and strategic ways.

The third point is based on the nature of the R&D process. The common view that the research, demonstration, and development process is a linear process and that strategic research kicks in at some predetermined point is much too simplistic. The cyclical nature of the process is evident each time we try to apply a discovery made in a simple system to a more complex system. Nowhere is this more evident than when a finding in molecular biology fails if applied to a development in biotechnology. The reason things do not work is that there is much we do not know about how molecules behave in the complex environment of a cell. A high level of sustained research in molecular and cell biology will continue to be strategically important to sustain a successful biotechnology industry. Examples of the strategic nature of academic research exist in other fields, and we must exploit them if we are to counter those pejorative sound-bite descriptions of academic research that continue to be used by the media. My second proposal, therefore, is to begin developing and communicating materials that clearly demonstrate the strategic nature of academic research.

These proposals do not involve easy tasks. But they are important tasks, and there are people who are good at performing them. Sustaining appropriate levels of federal support for science and technology while balancing the federal budget seems to be a task worthy of our best efforts regardless of the difficulty of the tasks. We should get to it.

11

Commentary: The Current Direction of the Federal Budget

Robert B. Helms

In this comment on the previous chapters, I would like to reinforce the points made regarding the impact of the growth of entitlement spending. Any discussion of the future of biomedical research must consider the potential for the federal government to continue its historical role of providing most of the financial support for basic medical research. The promise of new medical benefits from new discoveries in scientific medicine will continue to be attractive to members of Congress and political leaders, but their ability to support the further development of medical science may be severely hampered by other trends that will directly affect the federal budget.

To understand this threat, it is necessary to look at the federal budget and what is likely to happen to federal expenditures if current policies are not changed. For our purposes, it is important to focus on the distinction between discretionary spending and entitlement spending. Discretionary spending is that part of the budget that requires an annual appropriation by Congress. Spending for discretionary purposes is possible only when Congress has explicitly appropriated money for that purpose and this appropriation has been signed into law by the president. Entitlement spending, conversely, is based on the government's obligation to spend money for individuals who are eligible for certain benefits contained in several large entitlement programs. Such expenditures do not require an annual appropriation and are included in budget calculations based on actuarial estimates of the expected outlays. The largest entitlement programs are Social Security and Medicare, but numerous other programs provide benefits to federal retirees, Indians, veterans, and welfare beneficiaries that add substantially to the size of the federal budget. Entitlement spending is considered to be open-ended in the sense that total expenditures depend on the number of people eligible for each program each year and the cost of the benefits they are entitled to. These expenses can be reduced only if Congress takes action to reduce the number of people eligible for the benefit, to reduce the benefits to which they are entitled, or to reduce what the government pays for a given benefit.

The long-term trend in the postwar period has been for entitlement spending to grow relative to discretionary spending in the federal budget. In 1965, the year that Medicare and Medicaid were established, discretionary spending accounted for 65.8 percent of federal outlays. Discretionary spending had declined to 43.9 percent by 1985 and 35.9 percent by 1995 (Office of Management and Budget 1997). Reflecting the expected future growth of entitlement programs under current law, the Congressional Budget Office projects that discretionary spending will decline further to 30 percent in 2000 and 26 percent in 2006 (Congressional Budget Office 1997). The most recent reports of the Social Security and Medicare trustees indicate that both entitlement programs will grow at even faster rates after 2010, when the baby-boom generation begins to become eligible for these programs (Board of Trustees, Federal Hospital Insurance Trust Funds 1997; Board of Trustees, Old-Age, Survivors, and Disability Insurance Trust Funds 1997). This long-term situation is illustrated in figure 11–1, which shows both entitlement and discretionary spending and total revenues as a percentage of the gross domestic product. In discussing these projections, the Bipartisan Commission on Entitlement and Tax Reform pointed out that "absent policy changes, entitlement spending and interest on the national debt will consume almost all Federal revenues in 2010. In 2030, Federal revenues will not even cover entitlement spending" (Bipartisan Commission on Entitlement and Tax Reform 1995).

The political competition for discretionary funds will become increasingly intense. The analogy of a slowly sinking ship comes to mind. The rats are forced to expose themselves on the upper decks in a desperate attempt to compete for a declining amount of food and space.

By any historical standard, support for medical research has always been a relatively small part of discretionary funding in the federal budget. If the budget for NIH can be taken as our index of federal support, the president's recent NIH budget request of $13 billion for

FIGURE 11-1
FEDERAL OUTLAYS AND REVENUES AS A PERCENTAGE OF GDP, 1970–2030

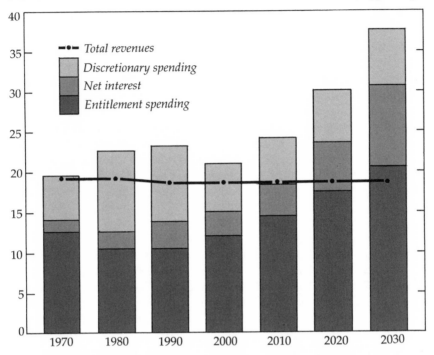

SOURCE: Bipartisan Commission on Entitlement and Tax Reform 1995.

FY 1998 represents only 0.77 percent of the total federal budget and 2.4 percent of discretionary funding. To illustrate the nature of the competition for these funds, a quick scan of the FY 1998 budget reveals the following discretionary programs that are similar in magnitude to the NIH budget request: space flight research at $13.4 billion and international financial programs at $15 billion. A similar scan of entitlement programs illustrates why entitlements are crowding out discretionary spending:

VA hospital services	$17 billion
Food stamps	$27 billion
Housing assistance	$28 billion
Supplemental security insurance (SSI)	$31 billion
Civilian retirement	$42 billion
Medicaid	$102 billion
Medicare	$207 billion
Interest on the public debt	$346 billion

91

In the public pronouncements of almost any member of Congress or any official in the administration, there are strong statements about support for biomedical research. But the ability to deliver on this support is severely challenged by the reality of the budget. In the absence of a willingness to impose large tax increases, the increasing growth of entitlement programs will continue to divert funds away from all discretionary parts of the budget, including support for biomedical research. The ability to use appropriated funds for basic research will be further hampered by the desire of politicians to support research on specific diseases rather than let such funds be allocated on the basis of scientific merit. Since few successful scientists are likely to become members of Congress, the only way to counter this political tendency will be to present more definitive research on the long-term scientific and economic benefits of basic research. This will not be easy, but it shares an objective that is valued by all scientists: the search for truth.

References

Bipartisan Commission on Entitlement and Tax Reform. *Final Report to the President.* Washington, D.C.: January 1995, chart 1, p. 9.

Board of Trustees, Federal Hospital Insurance Trust Fund. *1997 Annual Report of the Board of Trustees of the Federal Hospital Insurance Trust Fund.* Washington, D.C.: GPO, April 24, 1997; Board of Trustees, Old-Age, Survivors, and Disability Insurance Trust Fund, *1997 Annual Report of the Board of Trustees of the Old-Age, Survivors, and Disability Insurance Trust Fund.* Washington, D.C.: GPO, April 24, 1997.

U.S., Congressional Budget Office. *Long-Term Budgetary Pressures and Policy Options.* Washington, D.C.: CBO, March 1997.

U.S., Office of Management and Budget. *Analytical Perspectives. Budget of the United States, Fiscal Year 1998.* Washington, D.C.: GPO. 1997.

12

The Case for Dedicated Funding

Mark O. Hatfield

I would first like to set the scene on the question of biomedical research funding and its future. And I would like to go back two years because, at that time, there was a sharp shift in our ability to maintain the level of spending for the NIH. Efforts to reduce funding resulted in a prelude to disaster for biomedical research.

First, the president proposed a reduction in biomedical research for the NIH of 10 percent over a ten-year period. The House, controlled by the Republicans, was not going to be outdone. So Republicans proposed a 5 percent reduction immediately. The Senate, not to be outdone by the House in the budget resolution, proposed a 10 percent reduction.

The impact not only in that 1995–1996 budget year, but in 1997 and the escalation in 1998 and 1999 meant that we were truly dismantling our biomedical commitment. Action was required at the time. My colleagues and I called on the community to rally. We employed the Internet to get the message to about 12,000 recipients in centers of research, academic research, private research, and societies of the disciplines in science. From a Thursday when the message of "come to battle" to reverse this action went out, to a vote on Wednesday morning following, less than a week, we had an outpouring of the scientific community that I do not believe anybody had ever seen before. Scientists became political scientists for the day, and they recognized that this was a do-or-die situation.

Instead of reducing the biomedical research budget as proposed by the Senate Budget Committee, we were proposing to hold the budget steady. We won that vote, 85 to 14. It was the only amendment that reversed the actions of the committee during consideration of the budget resolution. Now that was a satisfactory and positive response to a crisis. In the end, the NIH received an 11 percent increase over the past two years.

Now, as we look at the year ahead for fiscal year 1998, we find, first of all, the president has proposed a paltry 2.6 percent increase in the NIH budget. The figure does not begin to keep pace with inflation.

Even worse are the out-year projections for 1999, 2000, 2001: spending would be less than a one-half of 1 percent increase. This effectively puts us back to square one, where the president started two years ago. At that time, although we had a Democratic president, it was a Republican Congress that tried to outdo the administration. It has been bipartisan posturing, in part, because there is no long-term funding strategy for the federal government's role in biomedical research. A meaningful long-term funding strategy will not rely solely on shrinking federal appropriations for medical research support. Alternative supplementary resources are a part of the solution.

Senator Tom Harkin, Democrat of Iowa, and I had proposed a trust fund during this same period to supplement federal appropriations but not to replace federal appropriations, not to be used by Congress to pick winners and losers but to reflect the same formula that is used by the NIH itself in allocating among its institutes. We had set aside a part of that trust fund to provide the director of NIH some discretionary funding to push through a threshold of some particularly promising projects. We also provided 1 percent for the National Library of Medicine because of our accelerating information needs and the additional costs of keeping pace with its dissemination.

We have tried various sources to finance a supplementary fund. First, we considered a 1 percent setaside on all health insurance premiums. Polls show that two-thirds of the American people support paying an additional premium tax if it is designated for medical research. We also considered setasides on managed-care contracts or setasides under Medicaid and Medicare.

One of my favorites is a tobacco tax, which also has strong public support if it is designated for medical research, whether it is a dollar or two dollars a pack. Canada has a three dollar tax on cigarettes a pack. Such a tax is not unheard of; it is not that innovative.

Our concept of alternative funding does not mean that it should be a replacement for federal dollars. Some believe that we could replace the federal funding program. I see no merit or wisdom in doing so. One of the few things the federal government does well is biomedical research and research in general—a true national defense priority.

Bear in mind, we also could look at the situation in matters relating to budget offsets to keep everything deficit-neutral as far as the increases are concerned. We must get by the droney, monotonous chant of "no new taxes, no new taxes, no new taxes," which is as irrelevant to our needs today as a balanced budget amendment. We have to have these budget offsets. No one wants to contribute to the deficit problem.

There are financing offset options. We have spectrums that we are auctioning off under the telecommunications act. In 1993, Congress directed the Federal Communications Commission to conduct public auctions for radio frequency spectrums and licenses, and in three years they raised $20 billion. In 1997, Congress also asked that 30 megahertz of spectrum be auctioned at an additional approximately $3 billion.

In Oregon, we have demonstrated the success of a voluntary income tax checkoff for medical research. We have supported Alzheimer's disease with $120,000 in our state's income checkoff system.

There are alternatives. We, in our effort of trying to put together a long-term strategy, should not be wedded to any one method. All should be debated. If there are other options or a combination of options, let us debate them. We need to get the debate going as to how we are going to supplement our commitment to biomedical research.

We continue to have unmet needs. Some are concerned that the goal of doubling biomedical research by the year 2002 could not be absorbed by NIH. Yet, 20 percent of grants that have been proposed to NIH and are considered worthy are funded today as against 50 percent of those grant applications a few years ago.

We also face a problem because we have Balkanized much in general in scientific education. When I started in higher education in 1949, we had sharp discipline divisions: for a sociology major, there was nothing in political science of benefit; for a political science major, nothing in sociology could be of benefit. Unfortunately, science has done the same to a great extent between what we call clinical and basic research. We know that fundamentally they are so interrelated that you cannot have one independent of the other.

As a former policy maker, I can say when you are facing a funding crisis and you come to Congress and say something to the effect that we have discovered a new gene, Congress will say, Well, that is nice. But if you say, We have discovered a new gene that leads us to the correction of a disease, then Congress is interested. It makes a difference in people's lives. That is an example of the interrelationship of basic and clinical research.

There is a continuum of science. And until we can get the scientific community to stand united on the bridge between the basic and the

95

clinical research, our case before Congress is not as strong as it could be. From a political point of view, the science community has to speak with one voice.

Ms. O'Neill has commented on the total amount of our science research funding provided by the federal government. There are eleven different categories or eleven different special listings for science research by the federal government. Defense leads the list. And this year it is $37.4 billion. Federal research dollars are also found in Health and Human Services, the National Aeronautics and Space Administration, the Department of Energy, National Science Foundation, Agriculture, Commerce, Interior, Transportation, the Environmental Protection Agency, and others.

This is an example of an increasing interest in a unified science and technology budget of the federal government, where we can monitor a comprehensive expenditure of research dollars. We would then have a better understanding of what our government is doing on behalf of science, science being interdependent, interrelated. As an example, consider the agricultural budget, which one would not think had much to do with the health of human beings, yet has produced nutrition research leading to vitamins and other such discoveries. We ought to have an interdisciplinary view of science fields rather than artificially putting it into categories.

These are important issues to consider. I am pleased that my former colleagues in the Senate have continued to place a high priority on biomedical research. Senator Arlen Specter, Republican of Pennsylvania, and Senator Harkin carry on the idea of a trust fund for research. We passed it in the Senate last year; it died in the House. The House has chosen a 1 percent setaside on the health insurance premiums as the funding source.

Senator Connie Mack, Republican of Florida, has introduced a resolution to double biomedical research funding. Senator Phil Gramm, Republican of Texas, has introduced one to double science research of the federal government. We are seeing a great deal of activity, whereas in the previous years only one or two members were active in this area.

This is the result of public support. Congress has broadened its base of giving leadership to science research in general, particularly in a new bipartisan way and from one end of my party to the other end of the party. I am encouraged that we have a moment to mobilize a united voice within the scientific community. The public has expressed its view: let us accomplish the great purpose of science: improving the future quality of life.

13

The Case against Dedicated Funding

R. Glenn Hubbard

I will focus on the issue of graduate medical education and clinical research in academic medical centers. Because my own work in economics really draws on tax policy much more than the economics of medical care, I will try to discuss the issue from a tax policy perspective.

I want to start with a story, generating a few ideas, and then go from there. Suppose an industry has a patchwork quilt of cross-subsidies that generate competitive problems and potential inefficiencies. Claims about deregulation of that industry, exposing sectors of its competition, generate fears of a lack of universal access; likewise, fears that the competitive process will discourage "outside" investment abound. I would argue that this is the discussion of this volume. My story, however, was about the telecommunications industry, in which cross-subsidies between local service and long-distance service have been generating inefficiencies. Some analysts have voiced concern that deregulation of the telecommunications industry would hinder telephone network development.

I could also reach much deeper into American industries—for example, banking, transportation, and my own industry, academia, which I will discuss here. I must have had bad karma in a previous life because I became a dean for a little while. In that capacity, I watched the university budget committee in action; its outcomes are not dissimilar to the kinds of cross-subsidies in medical research. I sit in the Columbia Business School, which pays into a cross-subsidy pool. I also sit in the Columbia Economics Department, which heartily laps up the same pool. In the university, we see the budgetary effects university-wide with the smallest tremor in the medical school.

In a number of industries—and in the important industry area of biomedical research—regulation has created cross-subsidies that engender difficulty. To illustrate the problems, let me start with a homily. In a democracy, public expenditures for clinical research or graduate medical education or anything else, for that matter, should be decided on a continuing basis within the political process. If we do not do that, we will not get the incentives for needed cost containment and reorganization in the medical research structure. Here I am focusing on academic health centers, but those other industries mentioned earlier are other examples.

June O'Neill and Philip Webre have discussed the budget backdrop, as did Senator Hatfield. I want to comment on the *B* word, the *budget* word, to indicate why it is difficult to imagine that the macro-budget environment ahead will not be a tough one.

The Congressional Budget Office has basically looked at two scenarios for 1998 for discretionary spending: freezing in real terms and freezing in nominal terms. The sticky wicket, at least from my reading of the CBO reports, is that something close to freezing discretionary spending in nominal terms will be required for the deficit overall to continue to fall after 1998. What does that mean? It would mean that holding discretionary spending to 1997 levels would lead to a loss of about a quarter of purchasing power by the end of the budget limit. That is a significant reduction.

How does one break down this discretionary spending, because, as Director O'Neill and Mr. Webre and Senator Hatfield pointed out, there are a number of components of discretionary spending? The defense component, which perhaps figures most prominently in the public mind, has already declined greatly in recent years. In the nondefense sector, it is by no means obvious that the health research and public health component, which is about 9 percent of total discretionary spending, could emerge unscathed. Caps on discretionary spending have, however, played a major role in our effort to control the deficit, and I would argue that adhering to them was made possible, in no small part, by this fortuitous decline in defense spending.

Now let us peel the onion back a little and return to the narrower issue of academic health centers and their financing. When one thinks of a medical school—Columbia Medical School, for example—one must think in terms of a complex of affiliated institutions. Think of the medical school at the center; the medical school is drawing on funding support from various levels: from Columbia University, the city of New York, the state of New York, and the federal government.

Affiliated hospitals—in this case, the Presbyterian Hospital, which is a fine teaching-research hospital—and affiliated practice plans of the faculty in outpatient centers also contribute resources. Indeed, for Columbia, the gross revenue of the faculty practice plan is actually an important line item in the gross revenue of the university as a whole. The faculty practice plans of medical schools are composed of doctors who treat the patients referred to the academic medical centers; these centers are divided into various groups along functional areas. In one sense, these functional areas are autonomous; in another sense, they are not. Deans, as they are wont to do, take their share. The term *dean's task* is a familiar one in medical schools: a dean might sequester part of the funds in faculty practices and assess 5–20 percent to give back to the medical school for educational purposes. Competition from other forms of health care providers, notably health maintenance organizations, is reducing potential cross-subsidies because the extra surplus to be allocated is lower than in the faculty practice plans. Contributions to a medical school from faculty practice plans and affiliated hospitals rose from less than 30 percent in 1980 to almost half by 1994. There has been a tremendous increase in the importance of this contribution.

If one looks at other areas of contribution in the medical school, pressures are evident. It is true that universities are continuing to increase tuition faster than inflation, though one must wonder how long that can go on; suffice it to say that there has been some pressure there. Even with the generosity of the asset markets, endowments have relatively low spending rules for most universities. Finally, research grants are under a great deal of pressure.

Hence, the threat of competition from HMOs on faculty practice plans is meaningful for academic health centers. Having said that, what could one do about it, in trying to shore up funding for premier research universities and academic health centers? Again, the key is to curtail the cross-subsidies, just as in the telecommunications example. In that industry, the curtailing of cross-subsidies has forced us to think about how one defines and pays for universal access. That is something with which Congress and the Federal Communications Commission are currently grappling.

It becomes more difficult to fund clinical research and high-cost academic health centers when the revenues from more practitioner-oriented activities are competed away. What policy issues are raised by this problem? One approach would be to pursue a goal of increasing support for graduate medical education in our nation's medical schools and research funds through a multiyear appropriations process and to make the pitch for greater support of our nation's medical schools. Another family of solutions is to somehow dedicate funds; trust funds offer an easy accounting example of how to do that.

From a public policy perspective, the former approach makes more sense—that is, trying to focus more on the continuing budget process, because the trade-offs in the budget process within discretionary spending are more transparent. That point returns to my earlier homily.

At the level of forcing innovation, that kind of a trade-off of forces—and I will try to be more positive here—encourages academic health centers to be more concerned about cost containment. A number of examples come to mind: creating one's own networks to compete against HMOs (and many academic health centers are launching into this business) and downsizing (an academic reorganization). Academic institutions are not necessarily the most efficient in the country. This is not a far-fetched notion hatched by economists. The Association of American Medical Colleges has itself said that before seeking broader tax-financed support, it is important to improve accountability in the eyes of the public about how efficient our academic health centers are.

A number of proposals aimed at graduate medical education and clinical research have surfaced in the 104th Congress. The idea is typically to guarantee some funds for medical education and to address the concern that the Medicare subsidies going to academic health centers may also be flowing to HMO providers who are not, in turn, performing research or covering a disproportionate share of patients.

In the Balanced Budget Act of 1995, which was vetoed by the president, Representative Archer incorporated a teaching hospital-GME trust fund, which would have included $13.5 billion over six years from general revenue plus transfers from the Medicare program. The Common Sense Balanced Budget Act of 1995, the blue-dog Democrat plan, would stop the current system of Medicare direct graduate medical education payments, indirect medical education payments, and so-called disproportionate share–uncompensated care payments from the calculations for adjusted average per capital cost (AAPCC) in Medicare. Seventy-five percent of those funds would be transferred to a trust fund for direct graduate medical education and the other 25 percent for deficit reduction.

The third proposal, from Representative Ken Bentsen, was the Medical Education Trust Fund Act of 1996, which is similar to the blue-dog bill just mentioned, with a few twists. Seventy percent of the current Medicare AAPCC payments would be returned to teaching and disproportionate share hospitals, and 75 percent of the direct and indirect payments would be placed in a trust fund to be distributed according to a formula that would be determined by a new entity, the National Advisory Council on Postgraduate Medical Education.

Fourth, the proposal by Senator Moynihan, the Medical Education Trust Fund Act, is a bit bolder. There would be free-standing legislation for a trust fund for medical education with average annual payments of about $17 billion between the 1997 and 2001 fiscal years. Where would the fund come from? The sources would be a 1.5 percent tax on all health insurance premiums, an assessment on the federal share of Medicaid expenditures for health care services, and the existing payments Medicare already makes in direct and indirect medical education payments; a separate account for medical schools would be established.

My concern about these proposals, which have the laudable aim of shoring up the financing for quite important medical research centers, is that they lack the critical element of competition in the budget process. That is, the elements that establish that incentive for cost containment and for innovation that are so important in many other deregulated industries, just are not there.

In thinking about these tax and trust fund schemes, we should consider a few principles. The first is to establish the research spending priorities, with reasonable cost-benefit analysis. As Frank Lichtenberg has said, that is not necessarily easy to do, but it is certainly the first step before one thinks about financing mechanisms: to decide what one thinks the commitment should be to this important component of research. Or, as Senator Hatfield had said, "Get the debate going, and the education process going."

Second, changes in spending on medical education and research should be decided on through the regular budget process. This important choice is among other important choices that the American people ask their representatives in Congress to make. Even if that is not done, any reform through a tax and trust fund system should have strong incentives for cost containment, reorganization, and innovation. Medical school accounts should involve competition for funds, not just historical allocations. We have to assume that innovation creates new players and bettering of schools, and we should not assume that historical allocations are necessarily appropriate. Finally, as a compromise between the annual fear of where we are in the budget process and a guaranteed trust fund, I would suggest a hard look at a multiyear appropriations process, which would give room to plan, while at the same time providing more frequent review.

PART FOUR

Intellectual Property and Open
Scientific Communication

14

Intellectual Property and Open Communication in Biomedical Research

Clarisa Long and Richard A. Johnson

Biomedical research is undergoing a paradigmatic shift from gene-centric biology to genome-centric biology that changes the way we think about biological innovation and genetic information. This new model asks fundamentally new questions, encourages competition in novel research strategies and in the development of new products, and provides startling new insights. The growing intersection of this new genomics framework with intellectual property rights is already profoundly reshaping the balance struck among the interests of biomedical research, private sector market participants, and the public good. The recent debates about the patentability of partial gene sequences, and their impact on the potential norms of scientific inquiry, are illustrative.

In the current context, intellectual property is about property rights to information. The policy challenges presented by a genomic-centered approach to biology in which information is the crown jewel greatly complicate the debate over the related questions of who owns what information and who can have access to it on what terms. This

The views expressed in this paper are the independent personal views of the authors and do not in any way reflect the positions or views of the American Enterprise Institute or of Arnold & Porter or any of its clients.

trend blurs further the faint, erratic dividing line between the public domain and proprietary interests.

Genetic Information and the Traditional Dilemma of Intellectual Property

Biomedical research creates numerous public benefits through genetic discoveries and new technologies that enhance economic growth and improve human health. Investment in genetic knowledge, however, depends on rights to future returns. The incentives created by intellectual property rights largely determine the pace and direction of this process, regardless of whether the research is publicly or privately funded. The available evidence suggests little doubt that proper incentives will allocate resources in the desired direction.

A system of intellectual property rights can provide incentives to innovate. By rewarding creativity, it encourages innovators to spend their time and resources in research and development efforts. It also stimulates the investment of resources needed to market the invention. By exchanging formal property rights protection for the inventor's disclosure of the information needed to reproduce the invention, such a system reduces the likelihood of duplicated efforts and increases the chance that further advances in technology will arise from the disseminated information.

The entire edifice of intellectual property rights is built around a simple dilemma: without legal protection not enough information will be produced, but with legal protection not enough information will be used. Economic theory hypothesizes that the private market will underproduce information because a producer cannot appropriate the full value of the information without protection (Ulen and Cooter 1996, 118). Information is the classic example of a public good. The cost of producing a unit of information does not vary with the number of people who will use it, and use by one person does not deprive another. From the standpoint of intellectual property rights, these two concepts can be expressed as *indivisibility* and *inappropriability*.

Information is indivisible or nonrivalrous, which means that it is undepletable; use by one person does not deprive another of using the same information. The information-producer incurs the same costs regardless of how many people use the information, the use of the information by others does not interfere with the producer's use, and the information can be used endlessly. This observation is not new. Almost two centuries ago, Thomas Jefferson noted:

> If nature has made any one thing less susceptible than all others of exclusive property, it is the action of the thinking power

called an idea, which an individual may exclusively possess as long as he keeps it to himself; but the moment it is divulged, it forces itself into the possession of everyone, and the receiver cannot dispossess himself of it. Its peculiar character, too, is that no one possesses the less, because every other possesses the whole of it. He who receives an idea from me, receives instruction himself without lessening mine; as he who lights his taper at mine, receives light without darkening me.[1]

Because information is intangible, harm to the information-producer arising from the failure or lack of legal protection is harder to quantify and thus does not create as much public outrage as theft of tangible personal property would.

The inappropriability aspect of this model states that in the absence of enforceable property rights, producers of information-intensive technologies will be unable to reap the market value of the information. The information itself has only a marginal value to the producer; the real value lies in selling it to the public. But sale of the technology reveals the information it contains to competitors and potential copyists, each of whom can copy the information and thereby recreate the value of the property at a price lower than that of the original producer. Unless enforcement measures allow the innovator to appropriate the value of the information, innovators will find the incentive to produce information diminished.[2] The information produced as a result of genetic research, however, does not fit entirely comfortably into this model: why was there no dearth of publishing in molecular biology and genetics in the years before the U.S. Supreme Court declared in *Diamond v. Chakrabarty* that genetically engineered microorganisms were patentable? The ability to appropriate the market value of a scientific invention is not the only factor motivating the producers of genetic information. To the extent that the law ignores those other motives, that omission will create dissonance within the scientific community.

The public goods qualities of this research suggest that without additional incentives the market will fail to produce the number of

---

1. Walterscheid 1995, 101–2 (quoting letter from Jefferson to Isaac McPherson, August 13, 1813). As secretary of state, Thomas Jefferson was on a board composed of the secretary of state, the secretary of war, and the attorney general that had the responsibility for examining patent applications. Patent Act of 1790, chap. 7, 1 Stat. 109–12 (April 10, 1790).

2. The U.S. International Trade Commission estimates that patent infringement alone reduces the annual investment in research and development by $750 million to $900 million each year (PhRMA 1996, 3).

creative and inventive genetic innovations that society requires. Unlike governments, private sector innovators must underwrite the costs and garner the gains from their investments in genetic knowledge. Private firm innovators, however, cannot capture sufficient returns from their invention or creation to justify the investment. Private firms must also estimate the appropriate levels of research under conditions of uncertainty and risk that exceed those of other investments.

The first big problem, therefore, is ensuring a sufficient supply of genetic information through research. Economists have found, however, that fostering more socially beneficial innovation does not rest solely with solving the public goods problem by tinkering with the incentives to ensure additional appropriability. As Peter Menell, among others, has pointed out, "Excessive protection for first generation innovation can impede later stages, thereby undermining some of the salutary effects of strong intellectual property protection" (1994, 2646).

The second overarching problem, often overshadowed by the initial issue of producing enough genetic knowledge, involves the diffusion or distribution of genetic information. In the end, a few widely disseminated genetic innovations may be more socially beneficial than many innovations with limited distribution. The problem manifests itself most acutely in trying to allocate fair compensation to the creators of valuable information assets, such as databases, while ensuring that other stakeholders have sufficient access to the same building blocks to provide the broader social benefits that the incentives have also been designed to provide. Researchers, for example, rely on more than 100 genomic databases available on the World Wide Web and many more available from proprietary vendors.

If the market underproduces information because of the indivisibility and inappropriability problems, the state can intervene to overcome the market failure and produce optimal amounts of scientific knowledge with policy measures Paul David has called "the three Ps: patronage, procurement, and property." The state can produce the information itself, subsidize the private production of information, or grant intellectual property rights (Ulen and Cooter 1996, 118). The Human Genome Project, the National Center for Biotechnology Information, and GenBank are examples of the patronage approach. Tax breaks and direct funding for genetic research are examples of procurement, and the patent system is a means by which the state grants intellectual property rights. In theory, the incentives created by proprietary rights are not necessary if the government provides enough direct support for biomedical research. Since the adoption of the Bayh-Dole Act in 1980, U.S. government policy has assumed that broad patent rights are a prerequisite not to achieve innovation but to ensure technology transfers from government labs to universities and on to the private sector.

An often overlooked point is that these policy prescriptions, from an economic perspective, are complementary means to achieve the same end—optimal amounts of discovery and innovation. They often are viewed, however, as conflicting policy approaches. Although the use of each may have other policy consequences that affect the desirability of their use, all three are substitutable; they are intended to solve the basic appropriability problem of genetic information that leads to the underproduction of such information by private sources without additional incentives.

Although the literature usually treats these three policy mechanisms as independent, the reality, at least in the field of genetic research, is that state production or subsidization of information rarely occurs without the invocation of intellectual property protection. Therefore, whether intellectual property rights can be granted for production of any particular kind of information is a factor that must be considered whenever we attempt to ascertain the efficiency of state creation of information. When we allow new technologies to be subject to intellectual property protection, or interpret intellectual property law in a new way, we make policy decisions that affect what kind of research is done, how it will be done, and how the results will be disseminated. Although attempts to gain intellectual property protection for the production of information may ultimately prove unsuccessful, information-producers nonetheless act with one eye on the intellectual property system.

Genetic Information and the Public-Private Distinction

Protecting Genetic Research. The two forms of intellectual property most relevant for the protection of genetic information are patents and trade secrets. Patents are the primary means of protecting the information generated by genetic discoveries. Patents grant the exclusive right to prevent others from making, using, selling, or offering to sell an invention for a period of what used to be seventeen, and is now twenty, years (35 U.S.C. §§ 154, 271 [1994 & Supp.]).[3] It should be noted that a

---

3. The legislation implementing the trade agreements resulting from the Uruguay Round of multilateral trade negotiations under the General Agreement on Tariffs and Trade (GATT), codified as Pub. L. No. 103–465, has altered the patent term from seventeen years from the date of issue to a term ending twenty years from the date of the filing of the patent application or, under some circumstances, the date of earlier-filed applications that are referenced in the later-filed application.

patent does not confer on the patentee the right to make, use, or sell; rather, it is the right to use the power of the state, in the form of access to the courts, to prosecute violators. In exchange for the right to use the power of the state to prevent others from making, using, selling, or offering to sell the invention, the patentee must reveal to the world in the form of an extensive and detailed public document the antecedent basis of the invention, a detailed description of the invention, all the information necessary to reproduce the invention, and the best means of using it (35 U.S.C. § 112 [1994]). With a few statutorily recognized exceptions, others who wish to use the idea can be required to pay the property rights holder in exchange for use of the intellectual property.

Not all discoveries are patentable. The range of patentable innovations is just a subset of all research outcomes. The committee reports accompanying the Patent Act of 1952 indicate that Congress intended to include "anything under the sun that is made by man" in the scope of patentable subject matter (Senate Report 1952; House of Representatives Report 1952). The operative language is "made by man": for an invention to be patentable, it must be new, useful, and nonobvious to one of ordinary skill in the art. Ideas, theories, mathematical algorithms, laws of nature, and the like are unpatentable. Patentable subject matter includes processes (including production methods, special techniques, and diagnostic methods), "compositions of matter" (such as microorganisms, enzymes, plasmids, cell lines, and DNA and RNA sequences), and new uses of an existing product and processes (35 U.S.C. § 101 [1994]).

The patent laws require that patentees reveal as part of the patent "a written description of the invention, and of the manner and process of making and using it, in such full, clear, concise and exact terms" as to enable others to recreate the invention (35 U.S.C. § 112 [1994]). Patent applicants who attempt to withhold vital information about the invention from their applications, in the hopes of extending the exclusive use of their application after the statutory period, run the risk of having their patents invalidated ex post. If competitors believe the invention is not fully disclosed in the patent, the competitors can challenge the validity of the patent before the U.S. Patent and Trademark Office (PTO) and appeal decisions by the PTO to the U.S. Court of Appeals for the Federal Circuit (CAFC). If the PTO or the CAFC concludes that the applicant misled the PTO when filing the application, such as by hiding relevant information, then the PTO or the court will invalidate the entire patent. The punishment for such "inequitable conduct," as it is known, is huge: patent invalidation. The anticipated value of the patent, therefore, is directly correlated with the incentive to act honestly when submitting the patent application. The more important the technology is, the broader the scope of the claims; the greater the antic-ipated stream of future revenue is, the greater the incentive for the patentee to be scrupulously honest and reveal all relevant information. Patentees will also know, ex ante, that a valuable patent will be care-fully pored over by competitors.

Under the "first to invent" system used in the United States, in which ownership rights are granted to the applicant who can prove prior invention (even if that applicant is not the first to file an applica-tion to patent the invention), independent discovery by a rival does not deprive a prior inventor of property rights, but it may raise the cost of defending the patent. Because applying for ("prosecuting") a patent is an expensive and time-consuming process, and because enforcing and defending a patent can cost patentees millions of dollars in litigation fees, patenting is a strategic decision.[4] Not all patentable innovations are actually patented. Sometimes researchers will choose for strategic reasons to release information into the public domain, or withhold it from the public domain, without seeking intellectual property protec-tion.

The incentives created by the patent system steer private research and development efforts away from basic research but also away from incremental improvements over existing inventions. Thus, the ability of inventors to reap gains from their own inventions, which is at the heart of the patent process, becomes stronger the more basic the inven-tion (Arrow 1962). As a result, universities and the government have traditionally performed much of the nation's basic research, while pri-vate entities do much of the development.

Applied researchers often accept the benefits of patenting without question, as well they might, because the genetic technology industry depends on, and has been built around, the patent system. Nonethe-less, the patenting system creates social costs in the form of the timing of data release, licensing and cross-licensing costs, and resources spent on litigation to protect the property rights created by intellectual prop-erty. In contrast, basic researchers often believe in the benefit of free exchange of information without private rights, but we will never know what therapeutic innovations have been lost for lack of private investment.

When an innovator cannot appropriate the monetary or nonmone-tary value from releasing the information contained in an innovation

---

4. The American Intellectual Property Law Association has recently esti-mated that the "cradle to grave" costs of prosecuting a relatively straightfor-ward patent in the United States range from $14,420 to $23,540 (AIPLA 1996, 446).

into the market, then the innovator has a strong incentive not to reveal the information but to use it as a trade secret instead. A trade secret is information that (1) "derives independent economic value, actual or potential, from not being generally known to, and not being readily ascertainable by property means by, other persons who can obtain economic value from its disclosure or use"; and (2) the innovator takes reasonable means to keep secret (Uniform Trade Secrets Act § 1 [1985]).[5] If the information contained in a trade secret is misappropriated, the holder of the trade secret may sue, but if the information is discovered independently by a second innovator, the holder has no recourse. Even if the holder of the trade secret believes a competitor may have misappropriated the information, litigation may still not be the answer because the holder of the trade secret will have to reveal the information in the process of proving his or her case.

The received wisdom is that if we wish, as a policy matter, to disseminate information expeditiously, patents are preferable to trade secrets because in exchange for the patent the inventor must disclose the relevant information underlying the invention. In genetic research, however, information has a short half-life. Information that is relevant and interesting today is passé tomorrow. If trade secrets are a thoroughly unsatisfactory means of disseminating information, patents are not an ideal way either. Even if information is disseminated through a patent specification, it can be stale by the time the patent document is published.

Genetic Research and Dissemination of Information. A number of factors determine the extent to which genetic information is disseminated. These include the absolute and relative costs of producing and disseminating the information, the incentives the intellectual property system creates to withhold information strategically, the ease with which intellectual property can be copied, and the incentives the scientific community has created.

Two kinds of costs are associated with creating information.[6] One is the cost of producing the information, regardless of how extensively it will be used. In genetic research, the cost of sequencing DNA represents a production cost. The second kind of cost is dissemination cost, which determines the costs of printing and distributing the information, whether through journals, the Internet, or some other medium.

---

5. Because the law of trade secrets has never been federalized, requirements for trade secrets and trade secret protection vary by state.

6. For a more thorough discussion of the economics of information production, particularly with respect to copyright law, see Breyer 1970, 292–302.

Suppose that the costs of disseminating the results of genetic research are decreasing because of technology, such as the Internet, whereas production costs are constant. This change can have one of two effects. In the first effect, more specialized scientific journals can be produced because production costs are spread across more consumers. In the second effect, if the market for consumption of genetic research results is saturated, fewer specialized journals will be produced with a larger circulation per journal. Whether technologies such as the Internet will create more specialized journals or consolidate existing journals will depend on the demand for genetic research information.

Publishing research results after filing a patent application does not affect the pending application. Nonetheless, patenting creates a disincentive to publish research results, even after filing a patent application, because such publication may reduce chances for a future, broader patent. These publishing delays create some inconsistency with traditional scientific norms. Norms within the basic research community would discourage keeping scientific discoveries secret while the application is pending. The intellectual property system, however, encourages innovators to get a head start in developing the applications of the new discovery before revealing the knowledge underlying the basic invention and thereby allowing competitors to benefit from the basic research. Such a delay in revealing that information is socially undesirable both because it delays the creation of second-generation products by other innovators and because it postpones the diffusion of the knowledge embedded in the basic invention.

Another problem facing a system of intellectual property protection in the age of high technology is the ease with which information can be digitized, copied, transferred, stored, and downloaded, all without detection. Traditionally, intellectual property, particularly patented property, was valuable because it created new tangible goods. A patented plow was valuable because of its tangible form, for example. But today, the value of most intellectual property is derived from the intangible information it contains. The cost of research and development for the products of genetic research is enormous, but once the product is revealed to the world, it is comparatively easy to synthesize or reverse engineer.[7] A copyist does not need to invest much energy or creativity in figuring out how to copy a patented product, because all the information needed to reproduce the product is contained in the patent document. The vaporousness of information influences the strategies that innovators use to protect their information, and indeed whether they choose to seek intellectual property protection at all.

---

7. Research and development expenditures on pharmaceuticals are estimated at $15.8 billion in 1996 (PhRMA 1996, 9).

Genomic research is different from most other forms of research in that collaboration is more essential than ever before. Genome maps, for example, are vital to research. In the case of the human genome, no lab can complete such a map alone, and such a map is essential to eliminate duplication of effort as multiple labs research the same regions of the genome. But maps are useful only to the extent that they are accurate and complete, and they can be completed only when information is released into the public domain. As Caplan and Mertz put it, "While a convincing case can be made for the value of patents in securing investment and attention for those who hold them, limiting access to portions of the human genome to a small set of scientists simply because they identified the sequences first is unlikely to lead to the maximal intellectual exploitation of this resource" (1996, 926). Critics worry that attempting to patent the products of genetic research will decrease the cooperation and collaboration between genome scientists necessary to create gene maps (Roberts 1991, 184). Critics also note the potential for conflicts of interest among scientists and are concerned that patenting will change the ethos of the basic research community (Anderson 1993, 300; NIH and DOE 1992).

Balancing Innovation and the Scope of Protection

As genetic research progresses and information is produced in new ways, new legal issues arise, the most fundamental of which is whether the intellectual property system can continue to maintain a delicate balance between information production and dissemination. Can the legal system create reasonably clear, bright-line tests determining whether the results of genetic research are subject to private rights of protection? In the absence of bright-line rules, how will the scientific community strike the balance between production and dissemination?

Patenting of DNA sequences is an example of an area in which the basic principles of protection have been worked out, although not without controversy. The basic techniques for sequencing DNA have been known for two decades (Maxam and Gilbert 1977; Sanger et al. 1977). The U.S. patent system views DNA sequences as "non-naturally occurring compositions of matter" that are patentable so long as their function is known and the inventor is not trying to claim them in a form that already appears in nature. Thus, the issues facing the genetic research community today are not whether DNA sequences can be patented at all but rather under what conditions they can and should be patented.

To obtain patent protection, the applicant must file an application with the PTO. Among other things, the application must contain a set of "claims," which describes the boundaries of the scope of property rights that the applicant would like to be granted. The application will typically contain more than one claim, and the claims will range from the general to the specific. The more general the language of the claims, the broader the scope of protection. The applicant and the patent examiner will then engage in a negotiation process in which the scope of the claims will be bargained down. Many applications never emerge as patents, and most of the patents granted never prove profitable for their owners.

The EST Patenting Controversy. In June 1991, the National Institutes of Health filed patent applications on partial gene sequences, or expressed sequence tags (ESTs), it had discovered (Caplan and Mertz 1996). ESTs are short DNA sequences some 150–400 base pairs long. They can be used as a probe to determine the location of a gene on a chromosome, but the sequence alone does not reveal the biological role of the gene or the reason a particular tissue expresses the gene. Although ESTs indicate that a gene exists and is active, or expressed, they do not always indicate the gene's function. The specification of the NIH's application disclosed more than just the ESTs, but it did not identify the full-length sequence of newly discovered genes, teach the biological activity of all the genes, or identify the proteins coded by those genes.

The NIH came under wide criticism for seeking patent protection for ESTs. Controversy arose over whether ESTs, or for that matter entire genes, could be patented when their function in the body is unknown (Adler 1992; Eisenberg 1992). Proponents of patenting sequences for unknown functions argued that disclosure of the sequencing information without attempting to patent the sequences might result in foreclosing "future patenting by anyone who discovers the full gene by identifying its function and . . . mak[ing] the newly discovered genes unattractive to private industry for use in product development" (Healy 1992, 665). The Association of Biotechnology Companies stated, for example, that it supported the NIH's decision to file patent applications on the ESTs "as a means to preserve its options on how to best utilize the technology for the public benefit" (ABC 1992a).

According to its statement, the NIH based its decision to file patent applications on ESTs on its desire to be able to transfer federal technology to industry by licensing the sequences if they were found patentable (Anderson 1994; Healy 1991). By filing patent applications on the sequences, the NIH was able to publish the results of its findings while preserving any potential intellectual property rights it might have. If it published its research results without filing patent applications on the ESTs, then under the U.S. patent statute it might preclude itself from filing patent applications on future discoveries involving ESTs because the later invention was either obvious or already in the public domain.[8] The NIH was concerned that such uncertain status of future patent applications would render the private sector less willing to perform research in this area.[9]

The NIH stated that it had decided to adopt a "pragmatic interim policy" of filing patent applications on the ESTs to resolve the issue of the degree to which the function of the DNA sequence would have to be known for a sequence to be patentable under the U.S. patent laws (Healy 1992). At the same time, however, the NIH was fully aware of the trickiness of the issues involved: it stated that it was amenable to an international agreement that publication of the DNA sequences would not preclude the ability, after further research, to patent the full gene, the products coded for by that gene, and the methods of using those products.

Opponents of patent protection for ESTs expressed both legal and social objections. According to their argument, because the patent application did not indicate the biological function of the sequences claimed, allowing the application to issue would allow the patentees to claim the rights to all products arising from the use of the gene. Some also noted that allowing patents to issue would run counter to the norms of science. In the words of Nobel laureate Paul Berg, "Patenting bits and pieces of sequence that are meaningless functionally . . . makes a mockery of what most people feel is the right way to do the Genome Project" (Roberts 1992). They also argued that allowing such protection would result in a deluge of applications flooding the patent office. Although the Industrial Biotechnology Association objected to the NIH's seeking patents on genetic sequences for which the biological function was unknown, it did not object to scientists in the

---

8. Under 35 U.S.C. §102 (b) [1994], an applicant is barred from receiving a patent on an invention if it was "described in a printed publication in this or a foreign country or in public use or on sale in this country, more than one year prior to the date of the application for patent in the United States." This one-year statutory bar creates tension between the incentives to publish research results and the ability to apply for a patent on the results of that research. An invention is also unpatentable if it is deemed obvious given the state of the prior art (35 U.S.C. § 103 [1994]).

9. See the testimony of J. Craig Venter before the Senate Judiciary Subcommittee on Patents, Copyrights and Trademarks; but see ABC (1992b) ("Whether future patent claims are obtainable . . . is not the concern of the NIH, which should not become engaged in schemes designed to ensure future exclusivity").

private sector doing the same thing (IBA 1992). The British Medical Research Council found itself in the odd position of criticizing the NIH for filing patent applications on ESTs, yet resorting to filing applications on approximately 1,200 of its own sequences as a defensive action. (Eventually the Medical Research Council withdrew its applications.)

In February 1994, the NIH abandoned its patent applications for the 6,869 sequences for which it had by then sought intellectual property protection after the PTO rejected the sequences on the grounds that their usefulness was unknown, among other things (Anderson 1994, 909).[10] (The patent laws require that an invention be "useful" to receive patent protection.) But the NIH was not alone in trying to patent gene fragments, nor has the patenting controversy ended with the NIH's abandonment of its application. The PTO reports that dozens of applications to ESTs filed by private sector firms are still pending. Indeed, because of difficulties involved in evaluating the patentability of this large number of sequences, the PTO estimates that it would take its biotechnology staff an entire year to evaluate the applications if it did nothing else (Marshall 1997). Although it has held hearings on the subject, as this volume goes to press, patent applications claiming thousands of nucleotide sequences continue to overwhelm the PTO.

The controversy over the NIH's attempt to patent ESTs raised numerous questions about the appropriate standards for patentability of DNA sequences (whether ESTs or otherwise), the proper role of federal technology transfer, and patenting strategies. In 1995, in an attempt to clarify some of the issues surrounding the utility requirement, especially as it related to inventions in the biotechnology and human therapy fields, the PTO issued its *Utility Examination Guidelines*. The guidelines stated that patent applicants should explain why they believe their inventions are useful (PTO 1995a 36,364); if the invention lacked a well-established utility, the applicants should assert a "specific utility" narrow enough to define a " 'real world' context of use" without further experimentation (PTO 1995b, 89–90).

In February 1997, a PTO official announced that the PTO had "decided to allow claims to ESTs based on their utility as probes" for larger DNA sequences (Vogel 1997). This decision only renewed the controversy over the patentability of ESTs.

Finding the Proper Scope of Protection. To date, the debate over the patentability of ESTs has centered on whether ESTs are patentable per

---

10. To be patentable, an invention must be new, useful, and nonobvious (35 U.S.C. § 101–03 [1994]).

se. The question that the intellectual property community and scientific community should focus on, however, is a different one: what scope of protection would be commensurate with the disclosed information?

The objective of the PTO is to avoid granting over- or underbroad patent rights to any particular invention. Overbroad patent rights provide the patentee with a reward disproportionate to the actual discovery, whereas underbroad patent rights do not adequately reward the patentee for making public the information underlying the invention.

As a scientific matter, a previously unknown EST is new, useful, and nonobvious. As a legal matter, under the PTO's *Utility Examination Guidelines*, it is new and nonobvious but not useful unless the applicant discloses a specific utility as a probe for a corresponding gene. To prevent an overbroad scope for protection, which would most surely occur if patents on genes were allowed to issue on the basis of ESTs only, the intellectual property system has chosen to set the hurdle for patentability higher than mere disclosure of the genetic sequence. By requiring that researchers disclose more than just a short DNA sequence to receive protection, the patent system institutionalizes the instinct of some commentators that simply sequencing DNA is not particularly inventive. Even if the PTO eventually allows patents on ESTs to issue based on their utility as probes, as it has stated it will do, the patentees will not necessarily get something for next to nothing; the resulting patent need not exceed the narrow scope of the EST described.

Another hurdle facing would-be EST patentees is the fact that a number of public databases of ESTs and other genomic information exist, two of which are GenBank and the Merck-funded database at Washington University in St. Louis. Release of such information into the public domain will often preclude the grant of private intellectual property rights to the same information. The existence of such public databases lowers the costs of conducting downstream innovation but also makes intellectual property protection for any particular sequence more uncertain.

At present, patentability standards to ESTs remain in limbo. Uncertainty in the standards for determining patentability is worse than a standard that overprotects or underprotects information. When the patentability of DNA sequences is uncertain—in other words, when researchers do not know, with a high degree of certainty, whether they will be able to exercise private rights over the embodiment of the information—the incentive to release information into the public domain is diminished, and researchers will hold their data as a trade secret.

Suppose a researcher knows that a DNA sequence is not patentable because it will be deemed obvious or will lack utility. Under such circumstances, the researcher can do one of two things: either keep the information as a trade secret or release it into the public domain. If the researcher would be unable to capture the commercial value of the sequence, or if such expected value is long-term at best, then the short-term benefits of releasing information to one's peers take on greater relative importance. Of course, the researcher may conclude that even if intellectual property protection is not available, withholding information is the better strategy because one can reach a patentable result faster that way or prevent a rival from reaching a patentable result. Which of these two strategies would prevail depends on the nature of the work, the predilections of the individual researcher, and the norms of scientific culture.

References

Adler, Reid G. 1992. "Genome Research: Fulfilling the Public's Expectations for Knowledge and Commercialization." *Science* 257 (August 14): 908.

American Intellectual Property Law Association (AIPLA). 1996. "Cradle to Grave Costs for a U.S. Patent." *AIPLA Bulletin* (March–April).

Anderson, Christopher. 1994. "NIH Drops Bid for Gene Patents." *Science* 263 (February 18): 909–10.

———. 1993. "Genome Project Goes Commercial." *Science* 259 (January 15): 300.

Arrow, Kenneth J. 1962. "Economic Welfare and the Allocation of Resources for Inventions." In *The Rate and Direction of Inventive Activity*, edited by Richard Nelson. Princeton: Princeton University Press.

Association of Biotechnology Companies (ABC). 1992a. *ABC Supports Filing of DNA Patents, Opposes Biological Diversity Treaty*. Press Release. May 17.

———. 1992b. *Statement on NIH Patent Filing for the Human Genome Project*. May.

Breyer, Stephen. 1970. "The Uneasy Case for Copyright: A Study of Copyright in Books, Photocopies, and Computer Programs." *Harvard Law Review* 84: 281.

Caplan, Arthur L., and Jon Mertz. 1996. "Patenting Gene Sequences." *British Medical Journal* 312 (April 13): 926.

Diamond v. Chakrabarty, 447 U.S. 303 (1980).

Eisenberg, Rebecca S. 1992. "Genes, Patents, and Product Development." *Science* 257 (August 14): 903.

Healy, Bernadine. 1992. "Special Report on Gene Patenting." *New England Journal of Medicine* 327 (August 27): 664–68.

———. 1991. *Remarks of Dr. Bernadine Healy at the Fourth Annual PHS Technology Transfer Forum*. November 14.

House of Representatives Report no. 1923, 82d Congress, 2d Session 6 (1952).

Industrial Biotechnology Association (IBA). 1992. *IBA Position Paper: Recommended Federal Policy Concerning Human Genetic Sequences Discovered by Federal Researchers, Contractors, and Grantees*. Washington, D.C.: Industrial Biotechnology Association.

Marshall, Eliot. 1997. "Companies Rush to Patent DNA." *Science* 275 (February 7): 781.

Maxam, A.M., and W. Gilbert. 1977. "A New Method for Sequencing DNA." *Proceedings of the National Academy of Science, U.S.A.* 74: 560–64.

Menell, Peter S. 1994. "The Challenges of Reforming Intellectual Property Protection for Computer Software." *Columbia Law Review* 97: 2644–53.

National Institutes of Health (NIH) and Department of Energy (DOE) Subcommittee for Interagency Coordination of Human Genome Research. 1992. Statement of January 3.

Patent Act of 1790, chap. 7., 1 Stat. 109–12 (April 10).

Patent and Trademark Office (PTO). 1995a. *Utility Examination Guidelines*, 60 Fed. Reg. 36,263.

———. 1995b. *35 U.S.C. 101 Utility Guidelines Training Manual*, August 22.

Pharmaceutical Research and Manufacturers' Association (PhRMA). 1996. *Opportunities and Challenges for Pharmaceutical Innovation*.

Roberts, Leslie. 1992. "NIH Gene Patents, Round Two." *Science* 255: 912.

———. 1991. "Genome Patent Fight Erupts." *Science* 254: 184.

Sanger, F., et al. 1977. "DNA Sequencing with Chain-terminating Inhibitors." *Proceedings of the National Academy of Science U.S.A.*, 74: 5463–67.

Senate Report no. 1979, 82d Congress, 2d Session 5 (1952).

Ulen, Thomas S., and Robert Cooter. 1996. *Law and Economics*, 2d ed. Reading, Mass: Addison-Wesley.

Venter, J. Craig. 1992. *Testimony of J. Craig Venter before the Senate Judiciary Subcommittee on Patents, Copyrights and Trademarks*. September 22.

Vogel, Gretchen, ed. 1997. "Gene Fragments Patentable, Official Says." *Science* 275 (February 21): 1055.

Walterscheid, Edward C. 1995. "Inherent or Created Rights: Early Views on the Intellectual Property Clause." *Hamline Law Review* 19: 81–105.

15

Commentary: The Move toward the Privatization of Biomedical Research

Rebecca S. Eisenberg

The authors of the preceding chapter have been so careful and responsible and nuanced in their presentation of the issues that I am at a loss to find fault with anything they have said. Instead, in the interest of provoking debate, I would like to use their monograph as a point of departure for looking at intellectual property in genomics from a slightly different angle.

One aspect of intellectual property in genomics that is highlighted nicely in the chapter and is particularly intriguing is that it provides a case study of continuing privatization of biomedical research. In this field, research of a sort that in an earlier era would likely have been performed in the public sector and widely disseminated is increasingly likely to be either performed in the private sector or privately appropriated as intellectual property by a public institution. This results partly from the Bayh-Dole Act and related statutes that, since 1980, have encouraged private appropriation of the results of government-sponsored research and partly from the emergence of private biotechnology firms that have found a market niche somewhere between the fundamental research that typifies the work of academic laboratories and the product development that typifies the work of researchers in private firms that sell end products to consumers. In effect, what is happening could be described as a privatization of certain types of upstream biomedical research that feeds into product development further downstream.

Somewhat ironically, this privatization is happening when bioinformatics and computer networking technologies make possible unprecedented synergies from the pooling of information from many sources. Thus, the familiar tension for the intellectual property system between using property rights to fortify incentives to generate information and safeguarding the public interest in widespread access to information is particularly acute in this context. We can see the dollars flowing into the genomics firms at the same time that we see the limits on disclosure of genomic information. The gains and losses from private appropriation are immediate and palpable.

Another set of concerns, also mentioned by the authors, is that a proliferation of intellectual property rights in the upstream stages of biomedical research could become a problem further downstream in the R&D cycle by imposing license and royalty burdens on the firms that are trying to bring new pharmaceutical products to market. Thus, intellectual property rights that restrict access to or raise the costs of research tools might present a net burden on the overall research enterprise that could be avoided by making more research tools available in a robust public domain. The decision of Merck to pay for the creation of an expressed sequence tag (EST) database in the public domain is a vivid statement of one firm's conviction that, at least in that particular case, downstream product development would be better served by dedication of research tools to the public domain than by their private appropriation. What is good for human genome sciences is not necessarily good for Merck.

While I have been mulling over some of these intellectual property issues at the public-private divide in biomedical research, my colleague at the University of Michigan Law School, Michael Heller, has been studying property rights in emerging market economies in the former Soviet bloc. Not until quite recently did it occur to me that, in certain respects, he and I are studying the same problem. With his permission, I would like to refer to his unpublished work.

In a forthcoming article in the *Harvard Law Review*, "The Tragedy of the Anticommons: Property in the Transition from Marx to Markets," Michael Heller considers why, even after several years of reform, Moscow storefronts often remain empty, while flimsy metal kiosks, bulging with goods, are flourishing on the sidewalks outside. He suggests that a significant part of the problem is that transition regimes have failed to endow any individual with a bundle of rights that represent full ownership of a storefront. Instead, they have created multiple rights in different entities that would all need to concur before an entrepreneur could set up shop inside. Partly as a carryover from the different allocations of rights that existed under the Soviet regime, perhaps aggravated by an unwillingness by reformers to face the political consequences of allocating fuller bundles of property rights to some holders of these rights while cutting off others, the new legal regime divided up rights in storefronts so that no single entity had the necessary bundle of rights to convey to an entrepreneur. As a result, different "owners," with different economic and political motivations, would have the right to sell, the right to lease, the right to receive revenue from sale, the right to receive revenue from lease, the right to determine use, and the right to occupy the property. Rather than face the enormous transaction cost burden of cutting deals with each of these owners and paying off any holdouts, many entrepreneurs choose the easier course of bribing government officials and the mafia to let them open up kiosks on the sidewalk.

At a theoretical level, when too many owners hold rights of exclusion over a scarce resource, it becomes difficult to put together the necessary bundle of rights to give anyone the privilege of using the resource, and it is underused. Economic waste results in what Heller calls "the tragedy of the anticommons." This articulation of the problem highlights the relationship to the more familiar tragedy of the commons that arises when too many owners each have the privilege to use a scarce resource and therefore collectively overuse it. Inefficiencies can result from a proliferation of insufficiently bundled property rights just as they can result from an absence of property rights.

The analogy between the Moscow retail trade and the U.S. biotechnology industry is not a perfect one. Yet, some similarities are worth contemplating in thinking about the future of biomedical research.

• Both involve the allocation of property rights in recently privatized exchange markets that had been dominated by nonmarket norms. In both settings, the previous nonmarket arrangements created expectations and senses of entitlement that will not disappear overnight.
• Both involve the allocation of multiple property rights to different owners who must be brought to agreement before anyone can effectively use the necessary property bundle for the benefit of consumers. A particularly vivid example of this in the genomics context is suggested by the prospect of patents issuing on gene fragments. Although it is not yet clear what scope of patent rights the Patent and Trademark Office would be willing to allow for the discovery of a gene fragment, one could imagine a serious genomic anticommons arising if it were necessary for a firm that wants to bring a therapeutic protein to market to obtain licenses to numerous gene fragments from different patent holders to market the product encoded by the full-length gene.

- In both settings, these property rights are held by heterogeneous sets of owners with different aims and different types of stakes in how their rights are used, beyond simply making money. One difficulty that Heller highlights for the Moscow storefronts is that the local government councils, workers' collectives, and regulatory committees that have different rights to the storefronts have different stakes in the current property regime and different reasons for holding out against assignments of their rights. Similar heterogeneities might be identified between the interests of universities, NIH, genomics firms, and pharmaceutical firms in cases where each of these property owners needs to come to an agreement before product development can go forward.
- In both settings, the applicable property rules are uncertain and unstable.
- As a result, the task of putting together the bundle of intellectual property rights that is necessary to put new products on pharmacy shelves is costly and fraught with uncertainty.

Obvious differences might give us hope that pharmaceutical firms will succeed where Moscow retailers have failed. The pharmaceutical industry is made up of experienced licensees of intellectual property with substantial resources for overcoming transaction costs. Nonetheless, the costs of obtaining multiple licenses can only be a drag on incentives for product development. At the end of the day, what keeps the pharmacy shelves stocked with new products is the profits earned by firms that enjoy an exclusive privilege to sell a new pharmaceutical product. We should be wary of allowing the development of a genomic anticommons that might interfere with the ability of firms to assemble the necessary bundle of property rights to reach that point. It remains to be seen whether one can sell new pharmaceutical products out of genomic kiosks.

Index

AAPCC. *See* Adjusted average per capital cost
Academia
    career timelines and, 30
    employment issues, 17–19
    funding, 98–101
    government and, 12
    Howard Hughes Medical Institute and, 24
    intellectual challenge in, 19–20
    medical education in, 22, 98–101
    medical research in, 14, 26–27
    peer review in, 28
    publication in, 43
    research choices in, 82–83, 88–89
    tuition costs, 12
    See also Universities
Academic health centers, 11, 22, 98, 99–101
Acquired immunodeficiency syndrome (AIDS), 15
Adjusted average per capital cost (AAPCC), 100–101
Africa, 15
AIDS. *See* Acquired immunodeficiency syndrome
Alfred P. Sloan Foundation, 70–71
American Association for the Advancement of Science, 80
Archer, William, 100
Asia-Pacific Economic Cooperation forum (APEC), 60
Association of American Medical Colleges, 100
Association of Biotechnology Companies, 115
Australia, 60

Barber, Albert, 4–5
Basic research. *See* Research, basic
Bayh-Dole Act of 1980, 43, 108–9, 121–22
Bentsen, Ken, 100
Berg, Paul, 116
Biotechnology
    diffusion of tacit knowledge, 47–51
    employment in, 53, 56 n 12
    excludability, 50
    patents, 47, 57–58
    property rights and, 5
    publication, 48–51, 52–55, 56–60, 112–14, 119
    "star scientists" and, 44–47, 51, 53, 57–60
    See also Genetics
Bipartisan Commission on Entitlement and Tax Reform, 90
Boyer, Herbert, 47
Bradshaw, Ralph, 3
British Medical Research Council, 117
Budget Enforcement Act of 1991, 77
Budget issues
    balanced budget, 85–88, 95, 100
    Clinton administration plan, 76–77, 79–80
    deficit, 75–76, 80–81, 98, 100
    discretionary spending, 4, 75–82, 89–92, 98
    implications for the future, 80–82
    spending cuts, 10, 82, 85, 101
    See also Defense spending

California. *See* University of California

125

*This book was edited by
Ann Petty and the Publications Staff
of the American Enterprise Institute.
The index was prepared by Julia Petrakis.
The text was set in New Baskerville.
Coghill Composition Company of
Richmond, Virginia, set the type,
and Edwards Brothers, Incorporated,
of Ann Arbor, Michigan,
printed and bound the book,
using permanent acid-free paper.*

The AEI Press is the publisher for the American Enterprise Institute for Public Policy Research, 1150 Seventeenth Street, N.W., Washington, D.C. 20036; *Christopher DeMuth,* publisher; *Dana Lane,* director; *Ann Petty,* editor; *Leigh Tripoli,* editor; *Cheryl Weissman,* editor; *Jennifer Lesiak,* production manager.